T0138936

Mastering Technical
Communication Skills

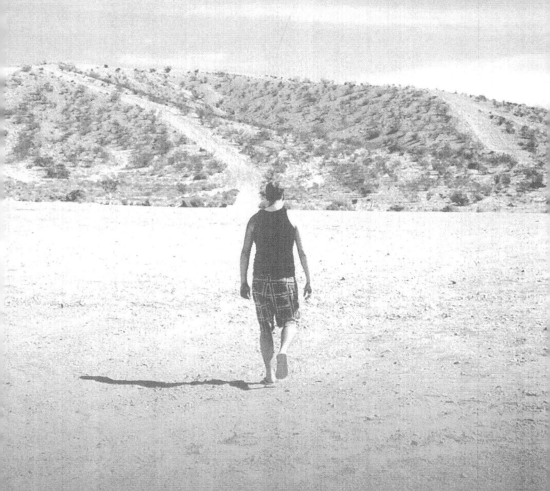

Mastering Technical Communication Skills

— A Student's Handbook —

Peter Wide

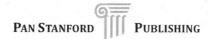

PAN STANFORD PUBLISHING

Published by

Pan Stanford Publishing Pte. Ltd.
Penthouse Level, Suntec Tower 3
8 Temasek Boulevard
Singapore 038988

Email: editorial@panstanford.com
Web: www.panstanford.com

British Library Cataloguing-in-Publication Data
A catalogue record for this book is available from the British Library.

Mastering Technical Communication Skills: A Student's Handbook

ISBN 978-981-4364-67-6 (Hardcover)
ISBN 978-981-4364-68-3 (eBook)

Printed in the USA

Contents

Preface

The word *mastering* in the handbook title is essential to the view of structuring an organization and involves a genuine effort to write an ambitious handbook. Students have, for a long time, asked themselves about the motivation to take a specific course, attend a seminar, or prepare a laboratory moment in their active student educational programs. As a professor, and for a period the dean of faculty at a progressive university, with a record of spirit and entrepreneurship, I am still astonished at the conservative structure of today's educational institutions. I have many times experienced a motivation problem by students for having just this specific knowledge, and to be really honest I have sometimes asked myself the same questions. A student's reluctance is, in many situations, a genuine doubt about the usefulness of a specific course or section of a course. Students are sincerely concerned about the quality of university courses given and the possibility to make use of the education.

The university structure and choice of educational programs, courses, and required knowledge are pretty much uniform in type, length, and content over the world. However, the benefits may lie in the possibility to evaluate, control, and compare education. But this structure also gives rise to a number of limitations, where values like alteration, innovation, and multiplicity are often part of a dynamics in an education that should reflect society in general and technological developments specifically. The need for a more flexible view of what a student should bring with him or her when entering society outside the university is of utmost importance when it directly will affect the student's ability to get a job as well as society to take advantage of new and fresh competence.

I have had an ambition to somehow, in a small step, redirect or rather complement the educational programs at the university level toward more future-oriented course alternatives. This would then also include interactions with students and their experiences. The young generation is known to be updated with all the technology trends actually pushing developments, for example, mobile phones, social media, and computer performance. To use past knowledge and trend analysis with today's experiences and create a starting point for estimating the required knowledge of tomorrow, that is, the period when a student is active on the market, has been my vision for educational development.

This handbook is considered one minor step to fulfilling the need for involving technology-driven knowledge with personal skills to achieve a student's requirement to be involved in a future society.

The strategy when writing this handbook has constantly been to follow the intention to focus on the primary concept from a student's point of view that easily can be read at the reader's convenience.

I hope that this handbook will be an inspiration source for anyone who has an interest in an emerging educational area of great importance. Although I foresee that students in various academic societies will frequently use this handbook as an inspiration source to further discussions and entrepreneurial ideas, other interested young people are welcome to use the advice in communication skills needed for an active life in society.

It is clear view that by mastering technology-related skills and using them as a way to improve communication and interaction with others, students will profit by increasing their ability to take part and act in a future society. The handbook is an introductory part of an inspiration guide that can be used by anyone, even if my ambition is to use this handbook as an important tool in a corresponding educational program at the university level.

I sincerely hope that as many students as possible get an opportunity to make use of this handbook and enhance their skills. The student will most likely meet the complex and, indeed, fuzzy expectations that a future employer may have, in order to be able to achieve highly skilled job opportunities.

Finally the content in this handbook may be condensed into the following three sentences:

Skill is about people meeting other people, mastering communicating ideas. This is the incentive that drives technology forward. I just encourage that combination.

Peter Wide

Chapter 1

Introduction: The Remaining Period of Your Life

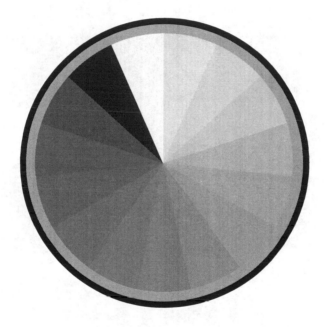

Good morning, Mr. X, and welcome to this interview for the position of project assistant at our successful, technology-driven organization, the Leading WorldWide (LWW) Company.

Mastering Technical Communication Skills: A Student's Handbook
Peter Wide
Copyright © 2016 Pan Stanford Publishing Pte. Ltd.
ISBN 978-981-4364-67-6 (Hardcover), 978-981-4364-68-3 (eBook)
www.panstanford.com

I am Mr. Harakumo, the HR consultant. Welcome to our multi-linguistic company.

[In Japanese] *I am Mr. Harakumo, the HR consultant. Welcome to our multi-linguistic company.*

[In Mandarin] *I am Mr. Harakumo, the HR consultant. Welcome to our multi-linguistic company.*

[In Spanish] *I am Mr. Harakumo, the HR consultant. Welcome to our multi-linguistic company.*

[In French] *I am Mr. Harakumo, the HR consultant. Welcome to our multi-linguistic company.*

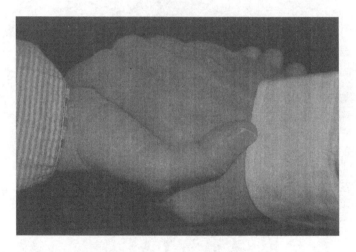

Figure 1.1 Two persons come in contact with each other.

Whatever language phrases are expressed in, there is often only one opportunity to exchange vital information about yourself.

A meeting between two people, for example as shown is Fig. 1.1, creates a situation in which both leave the meeting with increased experience. This experience can be new knowledge or modified information about the meeting itself or the person with whom one is interacting.

The next probable question from the HR consultant, Mr. Harakumo, will probably be, *Tell me about yourself.*

At this moment, the interviewer, Mr. Harakumo, is primarily interested in how you behave and how you communicate. Most likely he is certain that you have practiced this behavior for hours in your room and trained yourself on the presentation of responding to this specific question tens of times.

And, of course, you have prepared all your lessons before going for the interview. You are aware of how you are seen and perceived when you are giving the presentation (you have had your friends, relatives, or other persons comment on your performance and presentation technique so that you get an idea of how the interviewer will probably perceive you).

The initial moments of an interview or a meeting, when the persons involved are unknown to each other, are always of great importance. These moments are crucial for both persons to create a first impression. This first impression is then validated during the remaining time of the interview or meeting and helps decide the level of interaction during the conversation. This opinion is often difficult to change but can be more or less fine-tuned during the rest of the interaction, depending on the outcome of the interaction.

Therefore these moments of dual evaluation and opinion-making exploration are crucial for how you will be further considered and judged. Mr. Harakumo will, as expected, use his earlier experience of people's behaviors to focus on your specific behaviors and language presentation and compare these with your body language that, so clearly, communicates your intentions, meanings, and thoughts. For example, a relaxed, calm presentation in a smooth voice is not coherent with heavy perspiration and continuous fidgeting in your chair. This will most likely raise questions about whether you yourself are convinced about what you are telling Mr. Harakumo.

The conclusion is that you, for certain, will be examined in detail by the person sitting on the other side of the table, from your dressing code to your behavior during the interview.

In the very first moment, including the handshake (Fig. 1.1), the person you are meeting will form a first opinion about you. For example, are you "visible" for Mr Hamamatsu or is he not focusing on the situation Fig. 1.2). This validating process will then continue during the interview and can, during that time, be either strengthened or weakened; however, the opinion will usually not be too far from the first few seconds of an experienced impression.

Therefore preparedness before an important meeting or interview is wise. The only reason is you learn and become aware

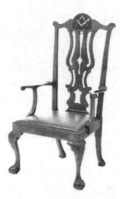

Figure 1.2 Mr. Harakumo does not focus on you at all.

of what signals you transmit to the environment. Only when you are aware of the signals you communicate will you be able to learn and maybe modify the impression and the significant picture you wish to present to the person with whom you are interacting, that is, how do you want others to perceive you?

In the communication process in an interview, there are at least four behaviors by which the interviewer will judge you. These four behaviors are relatively easy to be aware of and to adopt in your communication. They can easily be identified by asking a friend to listen to your presentation before the actual interview.

These four behaviors are:

1. You are according to the expected situation **representative.** Are you adapting to the specific situation and giving the impression expected in this specific meeting?

2. You are perceived as an **engaged** person.
   Is your body giving the impression you want the other person(s) to perceive? Are you stretching your body and having a positive smile on your lips? In other words, do you have a positive attitude toward the task you are performing?

3. You give the impression of having the required **knowledge**. Are you involved in situations in which you have enough knowledge? It is better to state that you do not have the

required knowledge than be trapped in a situation in which the other person discovers your lack of knowledge.

4. You give the impression of having **control** of the situation when communicating.
    Are your hands steady? Are you looking the other person in the eye when talking? Did you shake hands firmly with the person?

The four behaviors stating that you are representative, are engaged, have the expected knowledge, and seem to be in control of the situation will create a foundation that is most likely detected and evaluated by the person with whom you are interacting. These are excellent behaviors that will be perceived by others in your surroundings and will help you give a fair performance and get the expected or desired outcome from the meeting or interview.

The worst thing that can happen in a meeting or interview is that the person with whom you are interacting neither sees your qualities nor perceives your efforts to communicate your knowledge as well as your personality, Fig. 1.3.

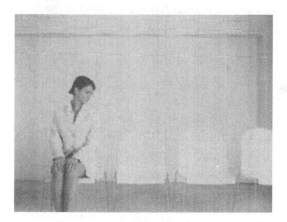

Figure 1.3 The person is not successful in communicating.

After the interview, when leaving the building, there is some time for consideration, Fig. 1.4. There are a few good rules to reach some conclusions as soon as possible after an interview:

- What impressions did you bring back with you?
- Did your perception sense something specific in the interview?

  ❑ *Smell*: Did you recognize any perfume or flower in the interview room?
  ❑ *Vision*: What did your eyes focus on when you were waiting before the interview?
  ❑ *Sound*: Did you notice any specific sound in the interview room?
  ❑ *Touch*: How was the interviewer's handshake (firm, soft, or a mix)?
  ❑ *Taste*: Were you offered coffee or tea and maybe cookies?

Your perception will, together with the interviewer, be added in your summary of that specific interview, and the outcome will be based on your earlier experience. The main issue is, however, to become aware of the total impression from the interview, and whatever the result, whether successful or disastrous, you will, as mentioned earlier, learn something from the communication. This experience will be added to your earlier experience, and there will be an increase in your total experience, that is, you will gain an increased amount of experience to be used the next time.

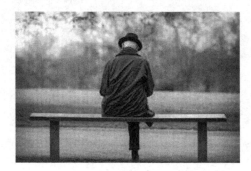

Figure 1.4 The process of reflection.

After an interview or a meeting, evaluating the interview or meeting is always a learning moment. It would be wise to try to answer the following questions after any interview or meeting:

- How did the interview or meeting go on a scale from 1 to 5?
- Were you satisfied with your performance?
- What was especially successful in your presentation?
- What did you learn for the next interview, meeting, or interaction?
- What can you change or modify about your communication?

The main recommendations that can be given in this situation are:

- *Good decisions come from experience.*
- *Experience comes from bad decisions.*

If managed to move forward to the next step in the employment process, it means you made good decisions during the interview, answered successfully on the questions and organized your presentation well. On the other hand, if you did not succeed this is a good opportunity to consider this interview as a moment to learn. Maybe, there is a possibility to request some feedback from the interviewer and be able to improve your interaction, behavior and presentation accordingly. Also, keep in mind that if you do not get any employment offer, the reasons could be depending upon different reasons, for example:

- the employment position was not appointed by any of the candidates
- an internship was suggested for the position; or
- a more qualified person got the job.

Chapter 2

The First Meeting with a Presumptive Employer

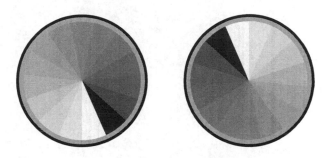

What types of job announcements will you see when it is time to take up your first job?

Are you prepared with the skills required?

Are attractive employers keeping up their higher demands as a natural selection phase?

These are strategic questions that the student of today most likely will have to handle before he or she faces the first job interview, Fig. 2.1, after academic studies. The student should also prepare himself or herself on how to compete with other students, as well as design a suitable portfolio containing a list of attractive courses and other experiences that will help fit the job requirements. How you organize your portfolio may be what *distinguishes* you from

Mastering Technical Communication Skills: A Student's Handbook
Peter Wide
Copyright © 2016 Pan Stanford Publishing Pte. Ltd.
ISBN 978-981-4364-67-6 (Hardcover), 978-981-4364-68-3 (eBook)
www.panstanford.com

other applicants and makes an employer choose you over others as a talented student with the most attractive track record. Or you may be chosen simply because you are just the most interesting person for that specific job!

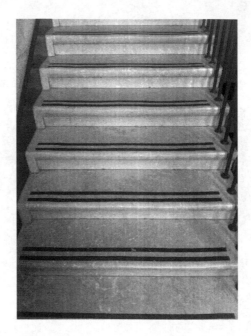

Figure 2.1 Climbing up stairs to the first interview is always a special feeling.

Each individual, whether he or she is familiar with the employment process, should be able to handle the first-interview situation in the best possible way. A student should be aware, in advance, of the expectations and prior knowledge that are valued in the recruitment process. This individually built-up strategy is of outmost importance for success in your career.

2.1 The Job Announcement

The following illustrative international job announcement is a nice example of a suitable, starting, initial type of attractive position. This position may be a goal for many students as their first international employment and the starting point of your specific interest and individual planned career.

The competencies and requirements for this specific vacancy announcement are as follows:

Competencies

Professionalism

The applicant:

1. Shows pride in his or her work and achievements
2. Is conscientious and efficient in meeting commitments, observing deadlines, and achieving results
3. Is motivated by professional rather than personal concerns
4. Shows persistence when faced with difficult problems or challenges
5. Remains calm in stressful situations
6. Is committed to implementing the goal of gender equality by ensuring equal participation and full involvement of women and men in all aspects of work

Planning and Organizing

The applicant has the ability to plan his or her own work to meet designated deadlines.

Communication

The applicant has good communication (spoken and written) skills, including the ability to draft routine correspondence.

Teamwork

The applicant shows:

1. Good interpersonal skills
2. The ability to establish and maintain effective working relations with people in a multicultural, multiethnic environment with sensitivity and respect for diversity and gender

Added qualifications for this job announcement are as follows:

Education: A high school diploma or equivalent is required.

Work Experience: Experience in general office support or a related area is desirable.

Languages: English and French are the working languages. For this post, fluency in oral and written English is required. Knowledge of other languages is desirable.

Other Skills

1. Good computer skills
2. Proficiency in standard computer applications for email, word processing, spreadsheets, and the Internet desirable

This specific, well-structured job announcement, which was found on the Internet, is specifically directed to the young generation of applicants for their first job application. This type of international job announcement is attractive to young people, and many students in the age group of 20–30 years will most likely apply. The students will certainly evaluate the possibility of fitting the job description. They will analyze the structure of the required skills and compare them with their own existing skills and experience before applying for the position.

If you have English and French language skills and a high school diploma and you feel comfortable with the rest of the required competencies, I would suggest that you send in an application for this position. Employers always have high expectations to find the best-possible, young, and enthusiastic applicants for a new job. However, two things may be of importance to consider here. First, after reading the text of the advertisement one or two times more and thinking about what the employer really wants the applicant to do, you might consider the work to be ordinary office work with minor responsibilities. However, it can be an excellent career start to work for a period in this position in this company. Second, the company most likely will find a person who will naturally fit into this position and maybe will also have the ambition to apply for further internship and work himself or herself up to other, more prestigious positions. There is a good possibility that the company, in the final evaluation phase, will consider 5 or 10 best candidates and follow a strategy to pick the best-available candidate among them who has the ambition to succeed in the job, as well as future ambitions to apply for other, more qualified positions in the company.

What is really challenging about this job announcement is the complex skills required. It would be of interest to an applicant to notice that the text, indeed, shows a touch of communicating the future direction. There is an impression of communicating the following rule:

A job opportunity of today is considering the job positions of tomorrow.

You may notice that the clear view and spirit in the job announcement fill you with the feeling of wanting to go ahead with writing an application. This moment of encouragement and impulsive inspiration is exactly what this employer wants to express with the text. The 13 required skills in the job announcement indicate the kind of circumstances that the applicant has to face. The employer's requirements are, indeed, ambitious and show the expected skills that an applicant must exhibit. Additionally, the job announcement can also be seen as a message of marketing strategy to the public that will read the text. The intention could, indeed, be to reflect the company's organizational competence level and the skills required in the company. However, the applicants, when applying for this position, should be aware of the strategic focus. Finally, it is the reader's considerations that will be decisive in determining whether an application will be submitted to the company's HR department or whether it will only be a dream moment of a possible job that exhibits both advanced skills and experience.

It may be interesting to know the origin of this illustrative job announcement. The online job announcement for a **team assistant** was a generic job announcement for an entry-level position published under the general service and related categories of the United Nations (UN) Secretariat in New York, Fig. 2.2.

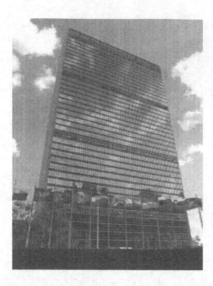

Figure 2.2 The UN Secretariat in New York, USA.

2.2 The First Interview

Being a student has certain implications. Student life is scheduled with many activities, both within school as well as in free time. Students have on a regular, daily basis a very hectic life, where an increasing number of more or less advanced courses is scheduled. Striving for added knowledge is the focus during this period. The eagerly awaited exam results should then be seen in the light of a continuously increasing number of credit points on the record list. The start of a new educational program in school or university denotes an important period that impacts a new student's life. The change in environment, when moving to a student dorm and getting a new social life with new friends, is indeed challenging but also very inspiring and inviting. The tempting new situation in a student's life is an intensive but often also a rewarding time.

However, your student life will at the final stage have an abrupt end when you suddenly hold the long-awaited degree in your hand. The past years of working time, maybe with minor responsibilities, that focused too much on individualistic performance suddenly change with an academic degree. The daily search for a classroom at a certain time to attend a specific course now suddenly stops. You have during some years learned from more experienced teachers, and now you have a fresh and updated education. The proof is now in your hand, and you may recognize that this university diploma will be an essential piece of paper that may help provide you with a career in a challenging, inspired, and socially oriented job. But being a student also consists of a continuous learning methodology and learning techniques.

The student time at a university is, in fact, a period when a student works on building a career that will provide him or her with a solid ground for future profitable recompensation. The skills that the student, with persistence and effort, builds up during this period are, of course, expected to pay back over time.

Students of today put enormous efforts into entering prestigious schools with brilliant reputations that will help them get better careers in future jobs. The goal is, at the end, to get a high-quality life. This approach is probably, partly, a right strategy because today's society is putting more emphasis on the university name than on the content of a student's track record. For most students this scenario is not an alternative. Since the vast majority of students are unable to choose or apply to prestigious schools, they may instead focus on other aspects that may play important roles in the strategy to find the best-possible educational and job paths in life.

Whatever skills a student may pick up and make use of can affect future challenges. The problem is that the student will be unable, in advance, to exactly know when combining different courses into an education will be an optimal solution for use in later interviews. However, the student has to be confident that his or her choices of courses and educational programs are the best-available options. A feeling of not choosing the right educational program will affect study time in a negative manner.

The most important factor in spending a number of years at a specific university is that you can always describe with pride in employment interviews, when meeting friends, and to your children that you enjoyed the study environment, the university, the dorms, the student friends, the teachers, and of course the courses taken, and finally the diploma ceremony, Fig. 2.3.

The advice given in this section is intended to start a moment of reflection and to use some time to carefully plan your dreams,

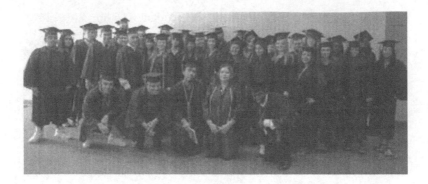

Figure 2.3 The end of university studies.

goals, and ambitions before putting them into a suitable educational program at a university that you have confidence in. The goals will help you find the best-possible educational program or, if the best option not is available, focus on the next-best solution. A good solution could also be to take extra courses in subjects that may be of certain value to a specific type of job. For example, when working in a multicultural organization a second, third, or even fourth language can be a competitive advantage, or when aiming to work in projects involving interaction with many coworkers, psychology courses may strengthen your educational portfolio.

Besides being more focused, today's student also has to remember that *what skills you focus on today can be very useful tomorrow, but you have specifically to influence your learning ambitions and choice of knowledge.*

You need to have a vision for the remaining period of life, or at least a well-defined action plan (or road map) of the coming occasions in the next one to three years. Then, of course, a dream of where you will end up in your career when you retire is always nice to add to the plans. I always state that when I am sitting in my chair in the elderly home and thinking back to my active life, there should be a multidimensional space for memories. There is, however, a risk of having forgotten the main parts of my history.

The main point described in this section is that if my defined action plan involves certain directions (road map), Fig. 2.4 I could at least state that I have tried to reach my goal by applying to the

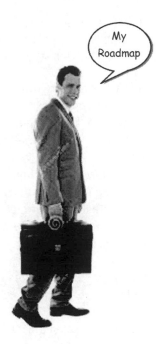

Figure 2.4 The content of the educational portfolio can be a competitive advantage.

expected extra jobs, moved to a proper location, and followed the expected course—that is, achieved the expected competence and experience.

2.3 The Employer's Agenda

The initial discussion so far in this section has been about how students can strategically act in a predictable and creative manner when they consider themselves to be at an important crossroads in life, as, for example, when aiming to find their first job.

Employers, of course, also have an agenda for employing the best-available workers who will create the best-possible combination of competence in the organizations.

A successful organization today certainly needs complexity and a complementary competence in coworkers, often with different backgrounds and experiences. Different languages and cultural variety are properties that are highly coveted when an international company is choosing complex skills to be integrated in its organization.

Therefore it is wise to sit down and think about the employer's ambitions, intentions, and points of view. These properties can advantageously be found on the Internet, for example, by searching or just by following the news. Also announcements are an excellent medium for publishing information about company policies, for example, about the environment, employees, or society engagement. Therefore, the announcement of a specific position has the goal of attracting young and fresh competencies. Usually it is up to the reader to find out the important issues in the text and estimate whether it would be rewarding to send in an application.

It is always worth to spend some time to put yourself in the employer's position, both in terms of the announcement text and in terms of what type of personality the company finds attractive.

- What issues is the HR person expected to focus upon?
- What qualities are requested?
- What personality, social-engaged, and team-working attributes are requested?
- What type of applicant is expected for an interview?

To conclude, what properties are essential for this specific position?

The question you will face in almost every interview is, why did you apply for this position in our organization?

The answer "Because . . ." is not an answer!

A good advice is to plan for questions that may arise at the interview and to foresee the process, Fig. 2.5. Try to figure out what type of quality the company is searching for. Does it expect to employ a hardworking, orderly, or creative person? Or maybe a complex personality that is stress resistant? Or a person who likes to travel, works hard, and speaks three different languages?

These questions are of strategic value and should be answered in order to estimate the chances of getting the job and reducing some extra work load, Fig. 2.6. By only applying for jobs that have a reasonably good success factor to not fail, at least in the beginning

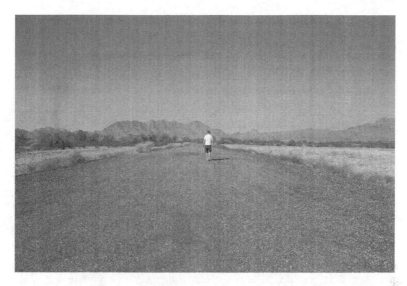

Figure 2.5 The road map is a technique to strive toward goals during a career.

of the interview process, the expected work load is kept within a reasonable limit. It is recommended that you send in an application only when you can communicate the main competencies that you

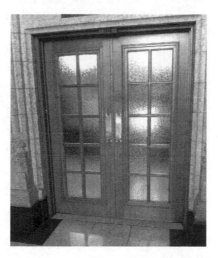

Figure 2.6 When entering the interview room you should be prepared and focused.

know the employer is requesting. Today it is not surprising that, in many cases, a vast majority of applicants do not consider the main aspects of the requirements in a job announcement.

Your job application must be proper and must answer the text in the job announcement. Do not try to make it more creative than necessary or be more visible than expected. Employers sometimes read several tens of applications, and often they read through the applications very fast and form an opinion about each applicant. There should be enough information in your application that notifies the employer about your acquired formal requirements and also about what type of person has written the application. Therefore, it is essential to know how to write an application. It should be formal in the sense that contact data, a curriculum vitae (CV), and maybe a personal letter should be attached, but as always the request in the job announcement will direct you as to how to write the application. The application should not be too long or too short and should contain relevant information about you and your essential history/ experience/formal education. There should also be a personal touch in the letter, for example, describing your interests, hobbies, etc. Keep in mind that some employers search social media sites for information about applicants, and you can easily be exposed and identified on social media sites. A strong recommendation is to separate professional issues and personal interests and your private and public information.

If you do not get a positive response to your application, it would be wise to get back to the contact person and ask for feedback. It is often essential to get feedback on why the application did not move further in the interview process and why you are not suitable for the position. There are always moments to learn more about how to communicate your competence and how other persons perceive the content in the text. However, in most cases, you will get informative feedback that will improve your next application.

After evaluating the feedback response from the company, you have two choices:

- To state that the feedback was certainly wrong, misleading, or discriminating.

    or

- To take the feedback into account and use the drawbacks to update and modify the next application.

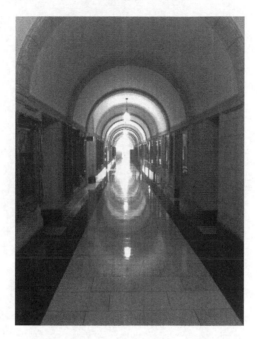

Figure 2.7 Longing for an attractive position.

By the end of the application process, you learn a lot, whether you get the position or you don't. With new experience, your next, hopefully modified application will be more adequate than before and focused on important matters, Fig. 2.7.

Chapter 3

Why a Student Should Be Prepared

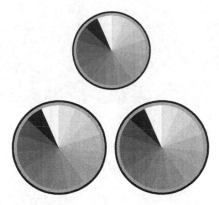

One of the most important questions today's students have to relate themselves to is, Is there any reason why a young individual of today not should be preparing for one of the most challenging occasions?

This essential issue may have a further impact on students' careers. The decisions made when young will most likely affect an individual's remaining active life in either a positive or a negative way. There is therefore the need for a sound and strategic action to plan for the next phase of life, a career. This plan, or map, has to be closely related to the choices, conditions, and possibilities that will be available for the kind of education, experience, ambitions, and other requirements the individual has. A carefully designed plan

Mastering Technical Communication Skills: A Student's Handbook
Peter Wide
Copyright © 2016 Pan Stanford Publishing Pte. Ltd.
ISBN 978-981-4364-67-6 (Hardcover), 978-981-4364-68-3 (eBook)
www.panstanford.com

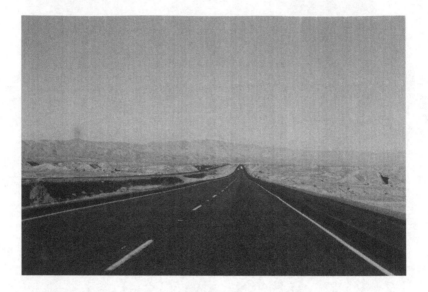

Figure 3.1 The choice of road leading to your expected career is yours.

of how to obtain a dream position as well as the next-best-possible career would be very useful, Fig. 3.1.

Let us find out what criteria are valuable and how the person you are interacting with thinks. Only then can you distinguish your competitors and find opportunities to communicate a message with a specific aim that if not controlled is at least understandable. A good strategy can be to go back and continue the discussion from the previous chapter.

The process of being well prepared is valid not only during the evaluation phase of employment but also when starting up a new company, working as a freelance consultant, or just continuing your educational/research activities.

There is a need to handle this process with respect. One possible advantage is to know your opponent, for example, in this case how the HR department thinks and acts as an organization and how the interviewer will influence the outcome of the interview. Will this circumstance affect your preparation, Fig. 3.2?

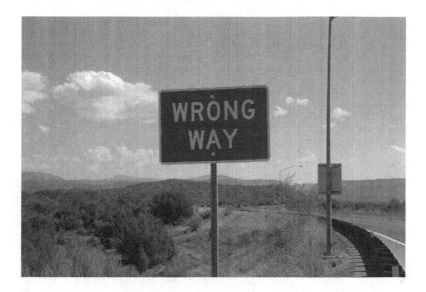

Figure 3.2 An individual needs to be prepared to make choices during the process.

The intention to write ambitious and highly qualified searches for employees is naturally not only a way to advertise an organization's goals and aims but also to establish the value of confidence in the market of human competence. This will, in the end, most likely increase the organization's attractiveness, draw the attention of well-educated people, and tell prospective customers that the organization is working insistently to employ young, skilled people. Therefore, the HR department has an agenda to fulfill the organization's goals and aims.

When you meet HR personnel at company presentations, job fairs, or job interviews, you will see the following agenda for "selling" their organizations when searching for new employees:

- Expectations in the organization are very high.
- The organization wants to employ highly qualified staff.
- There is an actual need for increasing the competence within the organization.
- There is an excellent working environment in the organization.

- The career is predictive and will be included in the plan.
- Opportunities are given.
- International experience is provided.
- The organization is intended for young, ambitious employees!

The general view is that the organization also has the same high expectations from the existing staff; however, this is probably not true. An organization of some critical mass has often an average of employees who, in many cases, behave as the population in general. It reflects the average of culture, age, and language composition as it often reflects society.

For example, an organization's staff may comprise individuals or groups who prefer to speak Spanish even if the company policy is English or who are fans of the local football club. Most likely the majority of employees share the views of the HR policy. But, in a company there are always individuals who do not sympathize with the company policy and seem to be in wrong positions or do not work in the direction of the company.

It is a fact that the human organization in a company often does not follow the policies and directions decided by management. That is why many dynamic companies offer their personnel over a certain age an option to end their employment at the companies. The offer can be financial compensation. This has been seen in many high-technology branches, for example, in the telecommunication industry, and the age limit where an employee is considered not to hold fresh competence anymore can be as low as the midthirties. It can be stated that this agreement between the individual and the company can have benefits for both.

A conclusion is that the recruitment process in a company also involves a communication window to the public that shows a high-skilled company that strives to get even better skills and improve its existing competence by complementing the existing staff with new colleagues.

But the underlining comment in this context is that *you may get a job offer even if you are not as competent as the profile described in the announcement.*

The advice on this complex issue is not easy. As a young student on the threshold of entering a career after a number of structured educational semesters, you should focus on general as well as special communication strategies. The general approach is to always be positive and enter new possibilities with joy and enthusiasm but also have the deepest respect for the different types of personalities you may meet in the employment process. You should also keep in mind that the HR staff always wants to do its job according to some given policy. However, in some cases you may also experience a situation in which the actual staff involved in a recruiting process may have its own opinion. This specific, related individual agenda may of course affect your strategy if you are trying to follow the HR staff's structure of questions. It may relate to preconceptions about the gender, age, or cultural conditions best fitted for a specific job.

This deviation from a job announcement can be argued on with regard to the company policy, services or products, and customers.

A quick and effective strategy in active communication, for example, in the recruitment process, is to show confidence and a sincere ambition to join the company of interest. A general knowledge of the company and its specific working tasks is always of great benefit.

Another issue that may be strategically valuable is your individual competencies. Investigate the similarities with the required profile and estimate how well you adapt to the profile. Normally you will not achieve 100% alignment with the profile. You have to do a simple analysis of what your chances are to succeed in the recruitment process. For example, how many steps after the first interview do you expect to take part in?

Some initiatives can be of use. For example, if the HR personnel want to show you the company site or invite you to lunch, a coffee, or a sandwich, there is also an agenda to establish your communication abilities and how well you perform in a social setting, for example, when having lunch with customers or simply taking a coffee break with your colleagues. These situations provide important details on how well you will act when representing the company.

This short introduction intends to highlight the expectations of the employer. These may be seen as insurmountable obstacles where you are continuously struggling to meet the given expectations, profiles, and demands in the recruitment process—expectations that focus on fulfilling all the imaginations, dreams,

Traditional process

Application arrive in time – and a receipt is received

Formal requirements are checked – according to job description

Read by administrator – often at the HR department

Placed into 1,2 or 3 groups – ranking the applications

Discussion internally – to find the best suitable candidate

Deciding a list of the most qualified applicants – final ranking list

The most attractive candidates are interviewed – normally only a candidates are chosen

Discussion internally – also including the department manager

Maybe new interview – a second interview /test phase

Offer to candidate – salary and benefits

Acceptance of job contract – formal signing of employment

Internet process

Net-based responding on a job description

Formal requirements are checked – according to job description

Administrator decides if candidate make personal / proficiency test

Test performed by candidate - often at home

The outcome of the tests decides if candidate are of interest

Interview often via internet

Offer to candidate

Acceptance of job contract

Figure 3.3 The different steps in the employment process are complex.

and expectations that you may have. This scenario is, of course, not true. The individual career is often a complex process with unique conditions, unexpected obstacles, but also many occasions that you never expected would show up. The dynamical interaction between you and an organization Fig. 3.3 in supporting your direction of career is, of course, a communication issue, which begins with the understanding that both parties are convinced:

- what the company representative is perceiving and you are communicating is common
- that you are the best available competence for a specific task profile, solving the criteria of fulfilling the announced job requirements

Coming down to the core, it is my belief that each student meeting the world outside the academia will consider his or her career as a means to *achieve a certain quality in life.*

This statement concludes this section.

An expected career is often ambitious, with high expectations, and sometimes it will be considered unfair. Nevertheless, a candidate can always relate that he or she did his or her best in every situation of the application process.

3.1 The Process of Being Prepared

The following section in this student handbook views the possible individual skills that a student may combine into an attractive competence portfolio of experience. The strategic decisions that have to be made when preparing for studies, part-time jobs, or access to important social networks are not optional. They are important to achieve a certain level of a single-minded combination of different skills in related subjects to achieve a master combination in communicating an attractive future curriculum vitae (CV). A CV is not just considered the main selling document when applying for a certain position. It is comparable with fresh food, that is, it is a perishable commodity and is your imprint for the specific moment when it is written or modified. A CV will consider a total specification that will be communicated to the environment. To master technical communication is to provide the environment with

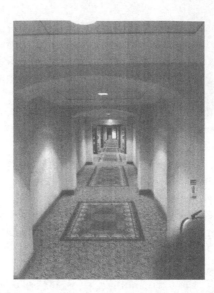

Figure 3.4 A fruitful conversation contains a number of consensus processes.

all techniques that possibly will help you make your individual and unique specification available at a specific time.

For a conversation to be fruitful for both parties, there is a need to get joint acceptance in order to enter the next level of understanding, Fig. 3.4.

A dynamical interaction is built upon a number of consensus covenants that need to be reached before a joint understanding can be considered. As Fig. 3.4 describes, a number of "doors have to be opened" before a consensus is reached. To be able to "open a door," the counterparty should accept the other party's level of understanding. For example, the candidate is suitable for the applied job, the competence is required, or there is a common approach in style, fashion, food, or whatever is discussed in the conversation.

If no consensus is reached in the communication process, it means that one or more doors will remain closed. This means that there will be a major problem to reach a consensus. This can depend on several reasons, for example, different personalities or facts presented unequivocally not reaching the expected level of predetermined requirements. This scenario can, of course, always

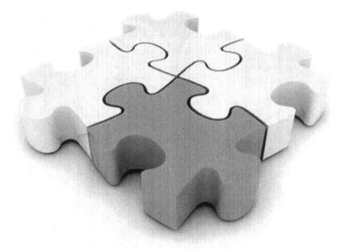

Figure 3.5 A successful conversation depends on an understanding of the communication information and relations of personality.

occur but will, in no sense, be a reason to modify the communication approach. This scenario will always be a possibility and has to be counted on. The recommendation is to learn from the situation and move on to the next job opportunity.

The performance of a conversation and the provided information are two main components that will be judged. These personality and communicated information issues, to a high degree, decide whether the dossier with your name will be placed in the "interesting candidates" pile and not be rejected in the initial stage, Fig. 3.5.

3.2 The Vision

An effective approach to envisioning your intentions is to write down on a piece of paper your intentions in life, describing a long-term, visionary ambition.

A vision is the overall level of intentions and the most successful goal, where the most ambitions and realistic conditions will be involved. The intention is to put up the level of a goal that, in many cases, will not be reachable. However, the main concept with a vision is that today it may be seen as an unreachable goal, Fig. 3.6 but

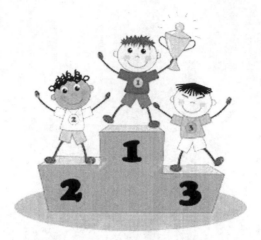

Figure 3.6 The vision should not be focused on a quest to become the best but rather to be good in a specific area.

tomorrow it may be a realistic goal, and the day after tomorrow it may be a reality, as illustrated in Fig. 3.7.

A vision is an intention about where you want to be in the future. But there are some conditions:

A vision does not need to have realistic expectations or demands.

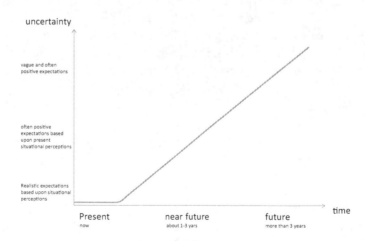

Figure 3.7 A successful visionary process.

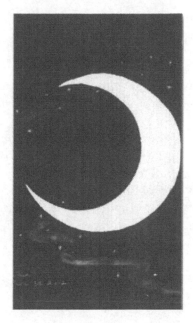

Figure 3.8 A dream to do business on the moon.

Further, it does not need to be related to time or even be measurable.

It is a dream, which is something to strive for, as illustrated in Fig. 3.8.

A vision is the process of striving for something and indicates the direction of and ambitions in a career in a few sentences. For a young person at the beginning of an independent and active life, this issue has many implications, for example:

- What are the specific highlights to go for in my specific career?
- Where do I want to reach in life?
- What positions, geographical places, and types of organizations do I covet in my expectations?
- What type of life do I foresee?

To understand a person's ambitions, it is essential that the communication be clear. A vision declared in a few sentences is an excellent start to further communicate in detail all the ambitions and conditions that every individual may have.

Some examples of student visions:

> *My intention is to become a rocket scientist. I will then focus on humanity and work to establish conditions for humans to live on other planets.*
>
> *I like fast cars. I have a dream to be an auto mechanic and work in an authorized car dealer of European sports cars.*
>
> *My ambition is to help people in emergency situations. I want to combine my ambitions with my dream to become a helicopter pilot. Therefore, working as a pilot in an emergency rescue service team is my vision.*

3.3 The Goal

To make a vision statement more understandable, with more details of how to achieve the visionary dream, it is essential to break down the dream into more understandable actions. It is a good strategy to decompose a vision into more comprehensible goals, as illustrated in Fig. 3.9.

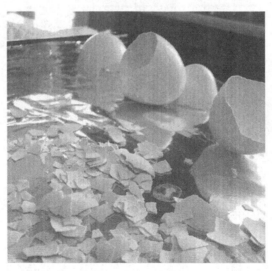

Figure 3.9 It is advisable to explore all the details in the whole picture.

The goals should be clear and simple. Each goal should also be realistic with clear time indications and with a possibility to determine whether it has been achieved at a certain time.

The following list shows how a goal is defined:

- A goal should be clear and realistic.
- A goal should be measurable—what conditions are needed to determine that the goal has been achieved?
- A goal should be defined in advance.
- A goal should clearly tell at what time it is reached.

Some examples illustrating student goals to achieve visions:

To become an engineer, I need a bachelor's degree in mechanical engineering from a well-reputed university latest by 2018.

To get work in ship construction, my plan is to get a degree from a prime national ship university before I am 26. I am focused on getting some initial practice and getting my dream job before 30.

My vision is to get a degree from a university program in emergency nursing and in parallel get certified as a helicopter pilot. My intention is to work as a pilot in emergency services directly after university.

I will learn to become an auto mechanic specialist within 3 years. Then I will actively apply for jobs at sports car companies. If I do not get an attractive job at a Ferrari dealer within a year, I will apply to a university and get a PhD degree within 10 years.

3.4 The Concept

The structure of a concept that reflects the momentary status of a situation or condition can be described in a *situational map*. A situational map can be described as a map showing the strategic or overall information at a particular time. It can also be seen as a snapshot of a person's available information. A situational map is a fresh-dated product, showing the situation of a person's collected benefits at a certain point of time. This map has to be updated each time it is presented to another person.

A situational map shows the current status of a person's experience, competencies, and other useful information. But it may also be seen as a description of the person himself or herself, for example, what intentions and plans does he or she have in life, what are his or her short- and long-term goals, and what type of personality is presented.

It is advisable to review the concept of a situational description in order to get specific and often unique properties into a situational map. These properties will, of course, be presented as positive conditions and as additive skills in communicating the person's competencies.

A situational presentation map is the latest updated version of presentation material that clearly communicates an individual's advantageous properties. It is recommended that you start with a general structure that involves the following parts:

Part 1: Future vision and aims. Provide a vision of your future status and how the map is designed to reach goals. This part of communicating is very important in clarifying your ambitions, mode of reality, and direction for a long period. It can be seen as information of:

- A personal view in life
- An individual vision with short- and long-term goals
- A plan for reaching goals, perhaps with an indication of certain activities needed to reach specific parts of the goals
- Validation of how realistic your vision is and how probable it is that it will be achieved

Write the future expectations with a touch of optimism and a visionary belief to work hard in a specific direction. However, they should also reflect some sense of realism in the process of getting results.

Part 2: Past history. A CV is a collection of earned knowledge, experiences, and competencies. The document is a description of life experiences and has, together with other skills, the status of a verifying document register. A CV should always contain information that can be verified, for example, a working certificate, a diploma, a language statement, or other merits.

An excellent example describing the design of a general framework CV or Europass CV has been established by the European Parliament and the European Council (Decision No. 2241/2004/EC) to create a European transparency framework for qualifications and competencies. More information about the Europass CV can be found at http://europass.cedefop.europa.eu/europass.

Part 3: Personal information. Personal information provides the reader with necessary additive information that is needed to make the expected evaluation and judgment concerning your abilities. The provided information should answer the following questions:

- What type of person are you?
- What social life do you have?
- What are your hobbies, interests, and other preferences?

A situational map should be a short description (preferably one to two pages), providing the reader with relevant information about you. This information may be of interest when establishing a value of personality. This issue is, of course, an important part when evaluating job candidates in an evaluation process for a specific position.

Chapter 4

Skills: What a Student Should Know

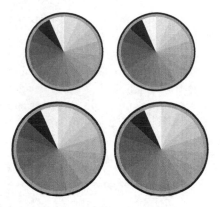

Students of today put in enormous efforts to enter prestigious schools with good reputations that will help them get good careers in future jobs. This approach can partly be a right strategy, because other aspects, too, may play an important role in the search to find the best-possible educational path. Acquired knowledge is something that is earned, and where this knowledge is acquired is of minor interest. Whatever skills a student may pick up and use can be of help in future challenges. The student of today also has to consider a strategic issue, that is, *what skills you focus on today can be useful tomorrow, but you have to specifically influence your learning skills and choice of knowledge.*

Mastering Technical Communication Skills: A Student's Handbook
Peter Wide
Copyright © 2016 Pan Stanford Publishing Pte. Ltd.
ISBN 978-981-4364-67-6 (Hardcover), 978-981-4364-68-3 (eBook)
www.panstanford.com

An individual vision is therefore a way of defining a strategy that will implement and direct the way to reach goals and focus on the actions taken to reach the visionary state of satisfaction in life.

4.1 Technology-Based Impressions

The young person of today has a certain style of living, where the dissemination of personality is an essential issue. In the image below the received mail is indicating that it has been sent from a cell phone. The unspoken message is that the interacting person has access to a "real time" communication ability that makes use of modern and maybe the latest available technology. What impression does this give to the environment? Well, in the wrong communication situation or with earlier wrong impressions, being available 24 hours a day might provide a negative conclusion. But in the right communication situation, for example, a fast and prompt reply to a meeting request, it will provide the receiver with the following impressions:

- The person has a cell phone (a smartphone), as indicated in the received message.
- The person is answering promptly because it indicates some sense of order when answering as soon as any phone call or message comes.
- The person is answering fast, indicating that the response is of high priority and therefore has been handled in due time.
- The person is acquainted with new technology and has already established a routine for handling incoming calls or messages.

These small details will always be read and coded by your friends, colleagues, or business partners. The individual style is important, and the way a person will build up his or her style becomes an advantage or disadvantage, depending on how the interacting person judges the situation.

The signal to the environment of being an extensive user of the latest technology trends in communication is a positive indication to successful companies that are eager to employ young people with the latest competencies who use high-efficiency technology. Using the latest technology tools will indeed reflect an ambition to be familiar

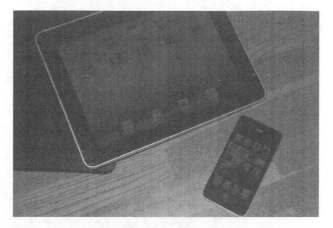

Figure 4.1 Communication tools often send a message to the environment.

with and apply efficient information media, as seen in Fig. 4.1. Also it shows that the person has:

- the ambition to communicate with others via a social network
- the ambition to search for external information on search engines
- a social life style
- an extensive technology-trendy personality

The trend can often result in a negative response from the environment if the user is sending personal information to other people, forcing them to listen to the communication, for example via mail conversations as illustrated in Fig. 4.2. This is an increasingly

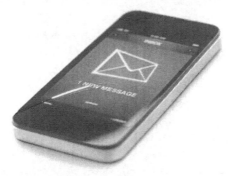

Figure 4.2 Received mail from a smartphone.

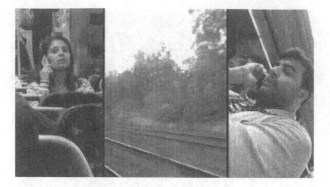

Figure 4.3 A person using public transportation and forcing others to listen to the phone conversation or music.

disturbing situation that everyone who uses public transportation has experienced at one time or another, as illustrated in Fig. 4.3. Imagine what message the person who creates this situation sends to the environment. What is the aim of this action, and what does he or she want to achieve?

4.2 Technology Skills and History

The skill of *knowing* and *knowledge* is a general basic structure for *self-comprehension.*

Knowledge is a normative perspective that has fuzzy boundaries that may differ between individuals, groups, branches, or cultural traditions.

Aristotle (Greek scientist, 384–322 BC) was one of the first to describe the phenomenon called *knowledge.* He separated knowledge into three parts with complementary skills:

- *Phronesis*—practical knowledge
- *Episteme*—scientific knowledge
- *Techne*—handicraft knowledge

Practical knowledge (phronesis) is nowadays considered silent knowledge that is referred to as the learning-by-doing concept.

Practical knowledge is often inherited, is difficult to describe, and refers to a traditional way of solving practical issues. To be a practical person is to know what action is morally right in a specific situation.

Scientific knowledge (episteme), according to Aristotle, contains only necessary knowledge, which is everlasting and unchangeable. This is different from the other two types of knowledge, both of which are changeable in time.

Handicraft knowledge (techne) is the base for technology-driven concepts. To use technology knowledge is referred to as the possibility to achieve a result from a starting point in a genuine understanding of predetermined principles.

Techne is placed between phronesis and episteme. Technology is knowledge when an engineer considers a control scheme, studies a drawing of a building, or writes a software program that is built upon advanced competence, that is, learned and exercised. When the engineer has to present the technology project (techne) in a meeting with investors, the human knowledge of practical sense (fronesis) is required. Additionally, when the engineer also refers to the latest scientific results, episteme completes all aspects of knowledge.

Aristotle's concept of knowledge involves a part of sound judgment together with a portion of reflection about the specific characteristics valid in the individual case that is called knowledge. All types of aspects are required to form a specific understanding of skills, experiences, and way to combine these into a specific knowledge.

The educational system of today is, in some sense, very similar, uniform, and simplistic all over the globe. We have to look backward in time, with our historical perspective glasses on, in order to establish a useful relation with historical landmarks that somehow connects to our present education. This may provide some sort of understanding of the existing educational system, which is based upon roots from the first university structures in Bologna (founded in 1088) or in the subsequent century at the universities of Paris, Salamanca and Oxford. This historical flashback may also provide a technology-based understanding of ideas, innovations, and commercialization that have pushed our society forward. The steam engine, penicillin, computers, etc., are illustrative examples of this (imagine how it would have been without these important innovations and the following commercialization). There are in most successful stories qualities of individuals who, with stubborn, progressive, and somewhat dissatisfied personalities, want to find innovative solutions that change the world.

4.3 Technological Breakthrough

The essential events of a technological breakthrough are improving both in time and in performance. Communication between individuals, groups, or globally has been impressive. The generation of people born during the 1950s has been through remarkable technical progress starting with the personal computer. The development phases were, in the beginning, fixed, heavy-weighted systems, followed by computers that were able to drag along in the first mobile versions. Then the real mobile and portable versions, laptops, appeared, which could be carried in a bag. The trend today is more and more to include computer functions into smartphones, which provide the freedom of multifunctional ability in a small phone.

The generation of the fifties will probably also experience and make use of the next phase of miniaturization technology in communicating functions. The trend nowadays is to make the communication systems more and more invisible and integrated with the individual. The development of small and increasingly smarter systems may in the coming decade be integrated with the body, for example, in the clothes or under the skin of a person.

Whatever solution is chosen, we can expect a dramatically technical development toward a more communicative ability in the future—a future where these functions will be used in an effective and useful manner to increase the individual ability to further improve the quality of life and be able to interact with other people whenever convenient.

All these new technology abilities have to include respect for individual integrity and personal adjustments. However, when predicting the future, especially technology trends, it is wise to take a historical view. The consequence of having more and more sophisticated technology interacting with an individual is, of course, a challenge. But the young generation will, as history has shown, have the best conditions to adopt and make use of new technology.

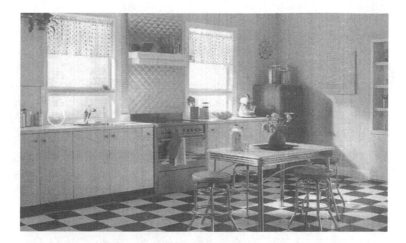

Figure 4.4 The modern kitchen in the modern house in the 1950s did not expect the use of computers in every single electrical product.

Young individuals are often eager to learn about new developments and adopt technology as per their needs and expectations. This quality could clearly be seen in advances in sending text messages using cell phones, called the short messaging service (SMS).

Look at the picture above, Fig. 4.4 and examine the type of innovation that the housewife was completely unaware of. This era was known as the expansion era, where families learned how to consume products and expectations to fulfill the needs of new technology to get a more sophisticated quality of life were enormous.

The consumption society was progressing in designing new and futuristic solutions that would manage to satisfy present needs. But society never reflected on the computer and the progress in communication abilities that each individual on the globe would see 50 to 60 years later. The information search on the Internet would have an enormous impact on society, which was totally unknown then.

4.4 Broadening of Your Knowledge

Since the future direction is not known, we may just have to guess, speculate, or use our imagination (or our vision) to estimate what type of knowledge will be useful in the future. The best-available recommendation anyone can provide in this situation is to always relate to oneself. With my perspective, goals, and ambitions, together with a touch of external influence and a great amount of information search, I should weigh the pros and cons in a specific circumstance. Since I will be best suited to make this decision on the basis of my ambitions, I can decide whether I will need extra knowledge in specific areas and skills in subjects that will make me achieve my goals. Then it is important to search for solutions that will bring me the additional knowledge by learning a foreign language, take advanced classes in environmental science, or learn cultural traditions.

However, the traditional view is to add some extra courses in business or economics in order to complement the existing educational program. These courses are often well known and accepted by employers and will be seen as a bonus when presenting your CV to a company.

But when you are finalizing an educational program, there may be a shift in demand by society. There is now an increased demand for more multicultural, broadminded, and wider knowledge integrated with the specialties learned in traditional educational courses at universities. The strategy is to take this knowledge into account when making an educational plan that will be the base of your CV. Future demands for other types of additional knowledge will always be an essential factor that, in some sense, will affect your CV when you apply for a job.

4.5 The Use of Knowledge

Knowledge is a source of freshness, defined by a certificate or a diploma that states to what degree the receiver has acquired the expected skills. Another factor that is of importance is the date issued, that is, when the receiver has completed the course. It is essential to verify whether knowledge has been acquired, by whom, and when. This is a natural procedure to establish a general system that acknowledges the competence worldwide. Therefore, the university system has been a reference for achieved knowledge.

The use of this knowledge can be communicated to people who are interested in your skills and experience. However, these organizations have a well-functioning system to evaluate different types of knowledge, estimate experience, and validate skills. The type of personality also reflects your ability to work as an entrepreneur in a major company, in a small business, or as a single company.

According to *The Concise Oxford English Dictionary*, an entrepreneur is defined as "a person who sets up a business or businesses, taking on financial risks in the hope of profit."

According to *The Oxford Paperback Thesaurus*, an entrepreneur is a "businessman/woman, enterpriser, speculator, tycoon, magnate, mogul; dealer, trader; promoter, impresario; informal wheeler-dealer, whizz-kid, mover and shaker, go-getter, high-flyer.

A traditional entrepreneur works singly and has no team inspiration, almost as a one-person company, as described in the definition above. The truth is that entrepreneurial work is available in a variety of positions, from single companies to big multinational organizations. An entrepreneur is a person who can find new innovation opportunities and develop existing business.

Entrepreneurial skills are a needed qualification that makes useful contributions in a great number of sectors of society, from technology to medicine and from social science to humanity, as illustrated in Fig. 4.5.

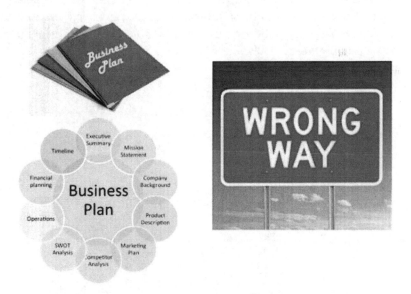

Figure 4.5 A traditional entrepreneur.

Today a complementing branch has emerged, from a traditional entrepreneur to an activity that implements a business involving the Internet era of information handling. "Infopreneurship" is a new, profitable direction in which individuals make use of the extensive information flow that exists. A business is then able to mine information and make a business case of delivering a specific service in providing the requested information.

An *infopreneur* is a person whose primary business is gathering and selling electronic information. The term is derived from the words "entrepreneur" and "information." An infopreneur is generally considered an entrepreneur whose business is to sell relevant and specific information by using the Internet as a source or media for selling. Selling information is a highly profitable way of using the global information process and is done by promoting development and marketing, as well as using blogs, websites, or e-books, articles, and active discussions.

An understanding of scientific information is essential to further understand the emerging knowledge that is available in libraries of universities and institutes. Scientific information comprises the research results disseminated by academic research bodies to other scientists, the industry, and/or the public. There is a general interest to get access to these information sources and to increase the knowledge of specific interest. These sources are often available to the public and are a valuable source for a student or ex-student to improve his or her knowledge.

Chapter 5

Mastering Time: What a Student Should Be Aware Of

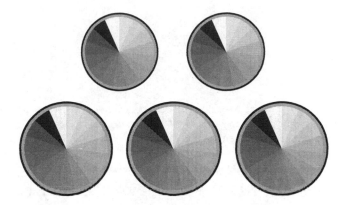

5.1 Time as a Physical Property

Time as a physical property is a unit of measurement and in the International System of Units (SI) is defined as the second. Since 1967 the definition of a second is *the duration of 9,192,631,770 periods of radiation that correspond to the transition between two hyperfine levels of the ground state of the atom cesium 133.* A second is abbreviated as s and sometimes also as *sec.*

Time is often viewed as a continuum in which events occur in succession from the past to the present (that's right now!) and

Mastering Technical Communication Skills: A Student's Handbook
Peter Wide
Copyright © 2016 Pan Stanford Publishing Pte. Ltd.
ISBN 978-981-4364-67-6 (Hardcover), 978-981-4364-68-3 (eBook)
www.panstanford.com

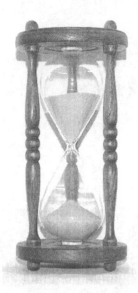

Figure 5.1 Sand flowing through an hourglass. When the upper part of the hourglass is empty, it means a certain time duration has passed, for example, one hour.

on to the future. This continuum can be seen as the sand flowing through a small passage in an hourglass, as shown in Fig. 5.1. The sand flowing is seen as the present time since the flow is continuous during a specific period, say an hour. The sand above the passage, which still has to flow down, can be viewed as the future, which will also happen within that hour. On the other hand, the sand already in the lower part of the hourglass represents the past, also part of the same hour, because it has already flowed down through the passage.

Time is a complex property that can be divided into two main categories, an external physical time represented by physical properties, for example, the time of day/night or the moon time between two full moons, and an internal biological time represented by the biological species' internal clock. Additionally, we have a setup time between different time activities in our social lives (Fig. 5.2).

Physical time is a moment of duration that everyone has to relate to and agree upon. It is a fundamental base in society and a common

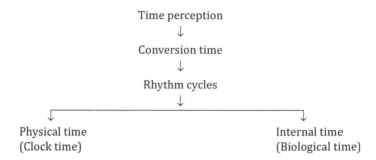

Figure 5.2 The human time perception as influenced by physical and biological times.

understanding of a general time that all people have to relate to when using public transportation, working in organizations, or just interacting with others. Physical time is set by different time zones around the globe, but the local time is still related to an external physical time.

Biological time is a time duration that we as individuals perceive. This time is often related to our biological rhythm, which depends on our heart rate. That is, we have a basic rhythm inside the body that depends on how we think of and perceive time.

The coherence between external and internal times may differ according to how we experience time and, of course, depends on our mood. For example, if we are tired, stressed, or hungry we may have a different opinion of the time duration.

Do the following exercise. Let's estimate a time of 23 minutes (23 min × 60 min/sec =1380 sec):

1. Set the timer on your cell phone to 23 minutes and start the stopwatch.
2. When you estimate that 23 minutes have elapsed, stop the stopwatch without looking at the elapsed time on your cell phone.
3. Calculate the difference in seconds between the stopwatch and your estimated time of 23 minutes.
4. Try to explain the difference. Was the deviation more or less than the objective time (on the cell phone)?
5. Repeat the exercise, maybe with a different time duration.

5.2 Scheduling of Time

Society is based on some basic structures. These structures help us manage our commitments without too much uncertainty, as for example a calendar Fig. 5.1. However, this organization requires that all involved parties respect and follow the rules and ideas of time. Time is a societal commitment that makes people get coherence between individual actions by having a joint agreement at the right place at the right moment. This is valid in most situations in daily life.

Let's understand this concept with the help of a simple but illustrative example. You book a flight to Canberra, Australia, for 5:00 P.M. (1700 hr), Saturday, September 3, 2014. This commitment between the airline operator and you (passenger), that the flight to Canberra will leave at said time on said date, has a dual understanding. The common understanding is that the airline operator will start the transportation to Canberra. It is, in some sense, agreed upon that the airline operator has a plane ready to start at that time on that date and you (passenger using the transportation) are present at the specified terminal before the departure time. There also are some hidden time constraints: the last call for entering the aircraft is a minimum time of X minutes before departure. The distance at the airport gate is approximately 12 minutes. Security control has a recommended time of 15 minutes but in special situations up to 30 minutes. If you do not check in online, using a cell phone or computer, you need an estimated 20

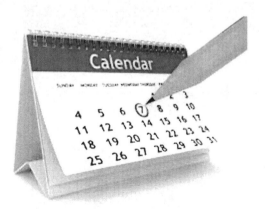

Figure 5.3 The importance of an active use of a calendar.

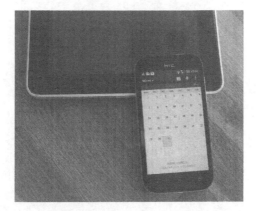

Figure 5.4 Cell phone planning.

minutes to check in at the terminal. Time scheduling at the airport is partly out of your control, so you should enter the airport building latest by 4:00 P.M. However, to ensure you catch the flight, it may be wise to add another hour to the time duration. The time schedule also includes travel to the airport. This time heavily depends on the traffic, time, and transportation vehicle. Therefore, it is up to you to control the available time constraints, time plans, and estimated delays to take appropriate actions in order to be in the right place at the right time. Otherwise, you will miss the flight.

The same strategic scheduling of time is recommended for every commitment you structure your daily schedule, for example in your mobile phone Fig. 5.4. For example, an interview meeting can have serious consequences if you are late even by a few minutes. The impression you will give is that you do not respect the other person's time. Additionally, you will give the impression of not being able to plan your own time properly. The main consequence, however, will be that you may be disregarded as a candidate in the evaluation process. The overall hint is to take time agreement seriously, especially with meetings where you might offend the other party by a delay.

5.3 Time in Business

Time is measured in seconds, minutes, hours, or even years. The human time perception is seldom in coherence with the clock.

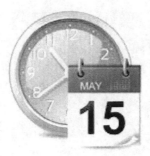

Figure 5.5 Communication in an organization mainly functions by time-bounded meetings.

Humans have a time dependence (perceptions) that, in some odd way, measures time that feels longer when one is bored or waiting for some special event to happen. On the other hand, time seems to fly when you are engaged in an activity you like or have an exciting meeting coming up.

Many people usually have a problem planning for time. It is always a battle to reach the airport, get to a meeting, or fetch children from day care on time. The deviation between the expected and the actual arrival time for an important occasion can, in some sense, also cause a problem for an individual's credibility with regard to his or her ability to work and function in an organization or society, Fig. 5.5.

This story is from real life:

It has been told that an inventor, an entrepreneur employed at a big company, had an important meeting with one of the major investors in the country. The investor has scheduled one hour for the meeting at the company. Unfortunately, the inventor was late, and upon entering the meeting room he started with an excuse: "I am 45 minutes late, but the transportation system is not working properly."

The inventor then spent some more time explaining the reason for the delay. The investor's team assured him that it was not a problem, because one hour was allocated for the meeting. The problem actually was now for the inventor and the company he

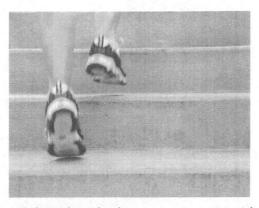

Figure 5.6 To be in the right place on time is an essential quality.

represented. The meeting was already delayed, and the inventor now only had less than 15 minutes to present his idea. This was a major drawback.

This example, in some sense, describes the culture of interactions between individuals or groups, Fig. 5.6. If you are late, do not expect that other people will compensate for that and prolong the scheduled time. People are very scheduled in organizing their ordinary working day and often do not accept any delays. Furthermore, there isn't anything more annoying than some being late for a meeting. This easily affects the meeting climate and outcome, too. It tends to create a negative atmosphere in the initial phase of the communication process.

The recommendation to young people is to also allocate enough time. In fact, double the estimated time of traveling to a meeting. Then, there will always be time for a coffee or to go to the restroom before the meeting, and you won't have to rush into the meeting room with a flushed face and heavy breath. Of course, in certain situations you do not have control over external situations that will affect your arrival and delay you. These situations hopefully occur seldom, and you don't have to begin with an "Excuse me" explanation.

Always keep in mind that someone—a person or organization— is paying money to get some amount of predefined work done. Someone is employed to actually do the job, whether it is in management or in storage.

The time value of work is money—the value of work for a given amount of money over a given period of time.

For example, $100 of today's money is invested for one year in work, and earning a 15% increased value by the work done will be worth $115 after one year. Therefore, $100 paid now for a certain task will be $115 paid back exactly one year from now. Both have the same value to the recipient, who assumes a 5% interest. Using the time-value-of-work terminology, $100 invested in work for one year at a 15% outcome has a *future value* of $115 by the work executed.

Time is money, and I have some time to offer.

5.4 Time Management

Time is something that everyone has; some just have less.

One often hears the statement, "I have no time." This statement is frequently used in society. However, time is a valuable gift that people can choose to use as effectively as possible. Time is also a property that can be planned and organized such that people can get a rich life and find meaning in daily activities.

To be resting on a sofa, listening to your favorite music is, at first glance, not an efficient use of time, Fig. 5.7. However, every person needs time to recover and to prepare for coming activities,

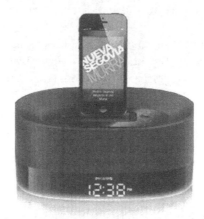

Figure 5.7 A positive relationship to time.

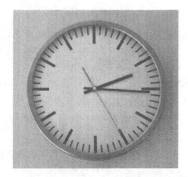

Figure 5.8 A negative relationship to time.

for example, an important meeting at the office the next day. People frequently relax and use music to help with specific thinking. Recovery time, as well as sleeping, going for a walk, training at the gym, etc., combines different activities with thoughtfulness. However, society will not accept that you spend hours every day in the office to lay back, shut your eyes, put on a pair of headsets, and imagine the structure of tomorrow's presentation.

There are different ways to approach a timeline.

A positive relation to a timeline will provide you with a few minutes to calm down and focus on the situation, whether an interview or a presentation.

A negative relationship to a timeline is, for example, to start a meeting with an excuse for being late, for example as shown in Fig. 5.8. This action may affect the meeting's outcome quite drastically.

People must consider the fact that things take time and concerns about time have to be taken in account. There are different types of time to note when scheduling a meeting. One main error is to define a proper time for discussion and conversion. This is often denoted as the setup time. The time for converting between two activities is a fragile reference, since this time is an individual time set. Therefore this time is frequently defined as too long or too short, depending on the individual's ability (internal clock).

The time and rhythm pattern is a fundamental concept in the life of a biological species. The cyclic internal rhythm that relates to time is an important part of the human calendar. Many of us make use of a rhythm in our lives. This rhythm has a short frequency of momentarily cyclic variations—daily, weekly, or even longer variations. The individual rhythm has a natural relation to heartbeat, and the frequency is a base for our living.

Rhythm, as defined in this case, is a frequency of events per second in Hertz, which is the official SI measurement unit of frequency. However, rhythm can also be related to the number of events per day or week or any other defined time length.

For example, if I have a rhythm of getting up in the morning at 7:00 A.M. and to get to school from Monday through Friday, I have a rhythm of five events per week. But if I suddenly have four exams per week and need to get up in the morning at 5:00 A.M. on Monday, Wednesday, Thursday, and Friday, this change in rhythm then disturbs my weekly rhythm and, as a result, makes me feel stressed. If I also have three obligatory meetings one week at my new job, it will certainly change my stress level and momentarily my rhythm.

Maybe this illustrative story can describe the life of our ancestors:

An Indian was going out to hunt deer for food for his family. He went into the forest in the morning, one sunny day, determined to catch a deer.

As he was sneaking among the trees, a rabbit went by. He let the rabbit go without disturbing the animal, because his intention was to hunt a deer.

Later, a duck flew by. He let the duck go without disturbing the bird, because his intention was to catch a deer.

Suddenly, a moose walked by, and like for the previous animals, the man let the moose go, too, because he was hunting for a deer.

As time went, he did not see any deer, and the day began to end. The man returned home at sunset and told his wife that he had hunted nothing.

Because he was out hunting for a deer.

This story shows that focusing on one task at a time was an essential parameter for our ancestors. This type of focus was still valid two to three generations ago, when our grandparents were young, and was a way of living.

The focus has now shifted from one single action at a time to multiple actions in parallel. This multiaction ability to keep up with

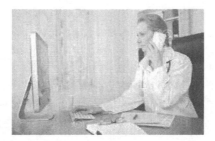

Figure 5.9 Prioritizing time is a person's own choice.

multiple processes at work is nowadays an advantage in many jobs as well as in family life, as illustrated in Fig. 5.9.

Today, the young generation uses cell phones as the reference external clock. This device, however, has some constraints. Wrist watches are in many cases functionality related to the battery, but cell phones have a battery capacity of maybe a day, depending on usage, as shown in Fig. 5.10.

The concept of time contains a focus on present, past, and future events. There are a number of past occasions that we are keen to remember, for example, birthdays, anniversaries, and also specific events, such as when you received an award in school, the first kiss, etc. Future time setups are mainly predictive in the short term, with a short and a long perspective, for example, the day when school

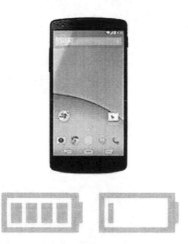

Figure 5.10 A smartphone with a low battery limits communication.

starts, the date of the next planned exam, and the time for the interview for a summer job. However, the start reference is, in many cases, the present. It is, therefore, important to put the present time in relation to the expected future or past time and to also involve the setup time, as mentioned earlier.

Here is an expression that is illustrative of the temporal and spatial aspects of life:

It does not matter where you come from.
All that matters is where and when you are going.
But it may be favorable to bring the history with.

Chapter 6

Technical Communication by Mastering Language: Essential Knowledge for a Student

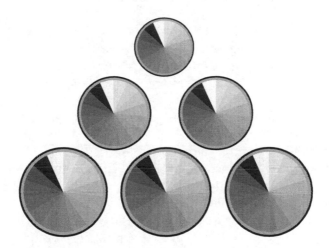

Language is among the oldest means of communication between humans. It is the basis of human communication.

There are four language skills that are important in interactions:

- Speaking
- Listening
- Writing
- Reading

Mastering Technical Communication Skills: A Student's Handbook
Peter Wide
Copyright © 2016 Pan Stanford Publishing Pte. Ltd.
ISBN 978-981-4364-67-6 (Hardcover), 978-981-4364-68-3 (eBook)
www.panstanford.com

Each of these four skills has its own nuances, and different communication situations require us to fine-tune each skill differently for convincing and effective communication. Fine-tuning words, melodies, and sounds is complex but can create delicate, powerful interactions.

A boy asked his uncle why he had only ve only one mouth to talk but two ears to listen. The uncle told his nephew that humans evolved this way so that they listen twice as much as they speak. Auditory senses are designed to listen not only by phase shifting to decide the direction of sound but also by effectively making use of auditory perception, which is approximately X% of the total human perceptual abilities.

Writing and reading abilities depend on two perception skills, speaking and listening, which are the primary functions of learning and writing or reading. An infant uses its listening ability and tries to mimic sounds in order to understand their meanings as the primary way to communicate.

An individual who masters the technique of speaking, listening, and analyzing the meaning of the other person's intentions will often be able to control the conversation. Your goal can, in some situations, be to convince a person or a group that your opinions are most relevant. In other situations, your goal may be to give a certain impression. Whatever your intentions, however, spoken communication is often a strong factor, when added to other human qualities, and can be an advantage in mastering a situation, for example, when applying for a job or presenting a sales concept or student work. The narrative task of language is an art that must be learned.

To take an active part in a conversation, we must also consider the output. To make a good impression, we should be active listeners and learn from others.

> *You will always learn from every conversation you participate in, whether it is a positive or a negative interaction.*

Spoken communication with a technical approach is related to both verbal and written skills and involves using these abilities in a language from a convincing, trustworthy perspective. Technical communication is, in some sense, very simple. Often, a subject is chosen and the goal defined—the content of, for example, a presentation and the type of audience and its general knowledge, interest, and level of learning needs are identified.

The goal is as stated above: to get your audience to learn as much as you want. Of course, if you make use of technical communication devices, your audience's understanding of the features, main concept, and solutions may increase. Here are some basic technical devices that easily increase the audience's learning abilities:

- Structure the content.
- Ensure everyone hears what you have to say.
- Use pedagogical vision pictures, for example, Microsoft PowerPoint presentations.
- Provide a clear message on the presentation's goal.
- Be convincing in what you say.
- Integrate a positive approach with your spoken and body language.
- Interact with the audience and be prepared to modify the presentation, if needed.

What is, then, characterized as a good oral presentation?

An inspired presentation provides the listener with increased knowledge by evaluating and maybe challenging his or her existing knowledge, resulting in new experiences.

I would just conclude that if your performance during a presentation gets positive feedback from the audience, it will inspire you. This moment is then a good learning moment. The comments, questions, clarifications, and maybe interruptions in connection to the presentation will inspire the audience to know more. It is positive when an audience member wants information that clarifies, exemplifies, or just adds to the content.

Every meeting will contribute to increased knowledge for the involved persons and result in increased experience. Even if you are involved in a conversation or listening to a talk that you feel is not a success, there will always be an outcome to it. This is also true for an interview.

6.1 The Communicative Language

Language is the most common communication tool that expresses an individual's mind in a complex, dynamic sequence. Language is used by all people of all countries around the globe.

Language is also used in situations in which no words should be spoken. How many of us deeply regret that we started some conversation or said some words in a specific situation?

A conversation between individuals can be seen as an impulsive, dynamic interaction that rapidly changes character due to the involved persons' ambitions to convince, clarify, or consolidate their own statements and confirm opinions. A conversation can also be like a game, when questioning the other person's arguments in trying to logically deduce what he or she means, aims, and thinks. The main objective is, of course, to get a view of the person's intentions. For example, what is he or she actually trying to say, or do I understand the logical-thinking path? What is the underlying message? Does the argument reflect my opinion? How do our arguments meld together, and in what parts do we disagree?

Communication between people is a complex, advanced process. We therefore need to understand the procedure of how we send out information and how we expect other people to accept and understand it. Then we can understand how people try to convince us that their arguments and opinions are the right ones.

6.2 The Spoken Language

A student has to perform on a number of occasions. This is a training process that involves the learning aspect—training to make presentations or lead a conversation. Whatever your ambition, spoken language is of utmost importance in order to communicate. The educational system should, from the beginning to the end, arm an individual with skills in the technical performance of communicating. An educational program should prepare a student using enough exercises so as to enable him or her to enter the business society with a professional mind and abilities to perform professionally. Also, there is an expectation that a person make use of existing technical devices to improve results.

Generally, a professional in business can be defined as a person who has enough skills in communicating technical issues and has also mastered general knowledge outside the specialist fields, can convincingly argue, and make conversations about related areas.

When communicating, speaking your mother tongue or a second or third language may take up a substantial amount of time from a working day. However, use of the official language is, in many cases, requested by the employer, for example, when presenting your work in meetings or representing the company to customers.

Speaking is an art. It is about convincing the listener, audience, or just a computer. It is a form of propaganda that you need to effectively do every day, often without any preparation.

The preparation of a presentation in spoken or written form is of utmost importance. Put yourself in the audience's shoes, whether in a meeting or a casual conversation with a person. You will realize that it is easier to achieve successful communication if you provide information in the format and content the listener expects to hear or needs to know. Instead of the presenter being a central point in the communication, trying to convince the listener of the presenter's point of view, the receiver of the information should be the primary target and focus. If the presenter becomes the focus of the communication, it often causes misconception that makes the communication fail.

A nervous presenter always attracts an unfair amount of spiteful attention from the audience. The increased adrenaline in the body causes the presenter to take unusual actions, for example, to speed up and talk faster than needed. A "normal" dosage of nervous behavior makes a presentation more active and effective if the person is able to control the behavior. The solution often used by people to control nervousness is to put a stone in the pocket and squeeze it before and during the presentation from time to time. This may have a calming effect and make the presentation more qualitative. Many professional speakers use this method when making presentations. Another suggestion is to not use the laser pointer when you are nervous, because you may highlight an incorrect point on the screen.

Since speaking skills are essential in many technical workplaces, the ability to understand and communicate technical information is highly needed. Reading and writing abilities are also of importance to effectively and strikingly interact with others, for example, in a team or organization. The ability to understand information maybe in languages other than your mother tongue is also sometimes essential. To communicate using spoken language smoothly and without misunderstanding, your words and sentences must be clear. An integrated understanding of communication is, of course, the best acquired ability in order to take part in an active communication and the flow of information without any or minimal possibility of misunderstanding.

In the present situation, when international organizations use English as the official language, there is a need for friction-free communication. Therefore, it will be an advantage if you acquire the necessary, basic knowledge of language as well as rhetorical skills. You can easily do this by taking extra courses in language skills at the university level and so strongly complement your portfolio.

6.3 The Listening Language

There are many aspects that can interfere with successful communication.

- It can be embarrassing and frustrating when your audience does not properly hear the spoken language if, for example, the technical devices are not working properly or if there is some disturbance interfering with the communication.
- As people get older, the ability to perceive sounds from the surroundings decreases.
- Many people do not take the time or, too often, seem to have insufficient time to listen to what other people are saying. For example, postpresentation questions can be valuable, since they not only provide a clarification of certain parts of the presentation but also provide a hint that you were probably not clear in those matters. Also, comments can enlighten the audience with complementary information, which can also be a valuable input for your next, updated presentation. Many speakers, instead, make short comments on the input from the audience. Also, due to limited time constraints, they often do not allow too much discussion postpresentation.

6.4 The Reading Language

Reading skills are an advantage. When learning a language, you read words or sentences, sound them, and finally pronounce them. Therefore reading when learning any language is an essential part of the learning process.

Many misunderstandings can be avoided by increasing reading skills. In an organization, there is always a risk of missing essential information when reading a text. Therefore, a strong recommendation is to read as much as possible about the expected target discipline of competence and to make use of the technical expressions that are expected in your specific field. For example, if you are aiming for a technical job or working in a technology company, you should understand the technical jargon and abbreviations used within the specific discipline, even in the marketing and human resources departments.

You can easily improve your reading skills by choosing relevant articles, books, or blogs from the Internet. The best results will be achieved by reading interesting scientific texts in the university or school library. By this, you will achieve a natural combination of language reading skills and specific knowledge, whether it is your mother tongue or a first foreign language or maybe a third foreign language.

6.5 The Written Language

Written text should have a structure that gives the reader an overall view and a recognizable organization of the text. The reader should be able to follow the content, and the flow should be both logical and informative. Also, being able to jump between text sections without losing the main message is valuable for the reader.

The structure of a text should be such that it is easily understood by the target of the information. The main message to be conveyed should be part of the information presented, whether it is a PowerPoint presentation or a short informational mail. You should make use of written language along with the different available technical communication tools to provide information to the audience in a presentable package.

The text should not be too long or too complicated to follow and must be written using easily understandable words. The sentences should be short and informative.

Effective written communication, at a minimum, contains the following sections:

- Background
- Main message
- Future aspects

This structure follows the past–present–future concept. The structure therefore is as follows:

- Past information: Providing a background
- Present situation: Providing the essential message
- Future intentions: Outlining future aspects

The scientific tradition of writing articles or reports varies between disciplines, but the general structure is as follows:

- Title
- Background
- Main message
- Summary
- References

The following scheme is more technical:

- Title and affiliation
- Abstract
- Background
- Main task
- Results
- Future aspects
- Acknowledgment
- References

The author of a text always has an intention with a written message. Text can be sometimes more convincing compared to, for example, spoken communication. Keep in mind that a writer usually has plenty of time to concentrate on every single word and create the "right impression" for the reader. Focus is also on clarification and structural organization of the information.

Written text can consolidate an impression through an intention, a background motivation, and analysis in a conclusion. Sometimes, the author also provides a reference list containing texts published by other authors. These texts are used by the author as references to strengthen his or her presented content and message.

The ideal approach in written text is to focus on the reader rather than the writer. (It is my intention to use this approach for this book, too.)

Chapter 7

Communicating Technology: The Essential Matters

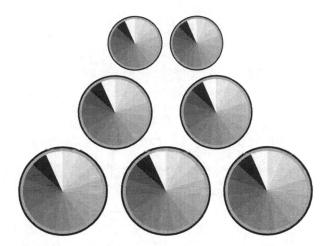

7.1 Presentation

Every professional individual continuously senses responses from his or her listener or audience, whether during a conversation or during a presentation. Every response can be easily noticed during an entire presentation. In fact, you can even get a feel just before the presentation starts and can then fine-tune your approach immediately before starting to talk.

Mastering Technical Communication Skills: A Student's Handbook
Peter Wide
Copyright © 2016 Pan Stanford Publishing Pte. Ltd.
ISBN 978-981-4364-67-6 (Hardcover), 978-981-4364-68-3 (eBook)
www.panstanford.com

Follow these strategies every time you are developing a new presentation:

- Determine the type of audience: technical, mixed, or nontechnical.
- Make the presentation on the basis of the audience knowledge or, more precisely, the average level cover related types.
- Ensure the presentation explains and clarifies to the right degree, making enthusiastic and learning impressions.
- Be prepared to skip a section or substitute one section with another due to the general interest.

During the presentation:

- Be active when presenting.
- Be positive.
- Be confident. Everyone should see that you know what you are talking about, and you will be seen as an authoritative person.
- Start with some personal remark, story, or impact to break the ice.
- Have a strategy during the presentation, depending on factors such as how the audience takes the information and what its interest level is.
- Prepare the content thoroughly and the presentation technique even more thoroughly.
- Keep a piece of paper with notes close to you in case of a mental blackout.
- If using technical equipment, understand the operation and use of the different devices.

After the presentation:

- Answer the questions as best as you can. Provide explanations that are of interest to the audience. Do not get involved in details that can be referred to later.
- Use the allocated time; do not use more.
- Conclude the presentation so that people know you are finished.

- Remember, there will always be a person who is an expert in the field, has more experience, and has more updated information. Accept this and state that this is your point of view and your preferences within the available specific conditions.

Keep in mind that the "nerd" in front of you or in the back of the audience who seems to be bored or asking weird questions can be your next boss.

Students continuously practicing various communication techniques will have probably already experienced some of the situations mentioned before, but there is always a need to concentrate on the mission of presenting an issue. Of course, you can use the given strategies as a reference for every new presentation.

Here is a checklist or road map that will provide you with valuable support and make your presentations even better. When asked to present something, clarify the following issues:

- Do you have time to prepare the material?
- Do you have access to technical equipment?
- Which type of presentation is expected: seminar, meeting group, or single person?
- Is the title or consensus of the presentation clear?
- Who will be listening, and what are their backgrounds in this specific issue?
- What are their interests in and expectations from this subject?
- What is the expected scope and time for the presentation?
- What is the expected additional information, documents, or pre-sent material?

7.1.1 *Visual Presentation*

A visual based presentation can be considered as the complete engagement with a vast information from the presenting person(s) that involves information provided as body language, spoken language, and behaviour. This means that the person presenting a visual-based material is generally perceived as the central point in the presentation. However, the main focus by the audience may be on the visual part of the presentation, e.g. the powerpoint slides. How the author is acting on the scene is closely followed by the audience, for example what type of shoes he or she is wearing to how he or she is acting or behaving. The other part of a presentation is often audio/visual, i.e. when the use of projectors increase the audience perceptual impressions by pictures, video files or story telling.

This type of presentation is important because the audience gives priority to visually perceived information, i.e. perceptual information on the screen. This means if you want your audience to perceive most of the presentation, then you have to use the visual informative material, complementing with an including spoken perception together with an illustrative and maybe gesticulating body language.

7.1.1.1 *The overhead presentation*

A visual presentation using a projector on a white screen is an improvement, considering the information effectiveness and also the involvement of our visual inputs. However, you should be aware of the following points:

- Only use summary text on the slides.
- Do not provide too much text.
- Do not mix or use improper colors.
- Add images or photos clarifying the text.
- Use the text as a support to the spoken language.
- Spend approximately two minutes per slide.
- Maintain contact with the audience by facing the listeners, not the screen.
- Follow the audience's interest in the presentation. If necessary, change the focus of the content by decreasing or increasing the time spent on some parts of the presentation in order to create a genuine interest in the given information.

7.1.1.2 *The computational presentation*

Use existing techniques to clarify the information being presented. If you want to describe the design of a chair, Fig. 7.1, for example, maybe an image of a chair, together with a proper description, will provide the right information to the audience, Fig. 7.2.

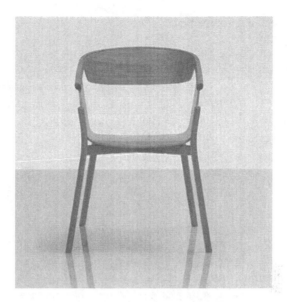

Figure 7.1 A picture of a chair is presented.

However, for a different type of audience, you may require other inputs to the presentation. If the audience comprises technology users, for example, engineers and designers, or users with minor technical skills, a software model can more illustratively describe the chair and its design.

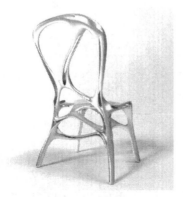

Figure 7.2 Software modeling of a virtual chair.

7.1.2 *Oral Presentation*

Now let's focus on the speaker's performance. The following list of items should be in every speaker's mind all the time. The best way to be aware of these items is to let a friend or student friend listen to you when you practice your presentation. An objective response based on these items can provide you with useful ideas to modify and learn new strategic steps toward a more accomplished presentation.

These suggestions will improve your oral skills in a person-to-person presentation as well as a meeting or seminar with an audience:

- Can people hear you clearly? Do you adjust your voice according to the number of audience members, the room's design, light conditions, etc.?
- Do you vary your voice in tone or volume and use body movements to express different parts of the presentation?
- Do you optimize the timing, not talking too fast or too slow?
- Do you portray active, positive authority and professional communication when entering the room, walking, standing, or even sitting in front of the listeners?
- How do you generally behave?
- What is your charisma, and what is the type of charisma you want to portray?

7.1.3 *Auditory Aspects*

To get the best-possible results out of your presentation, focus on the listener. The main purpose of a talk is to communicate. Whether the communication has a mission or it does not, the result will always provide information. Mostly, if the information has some value for the listener, the meeting has been positive.

To get the listener's point of view, there are some important steps to follow. The speaker may be prepared for things that he or she failed to get through and get a golden opportunity to learn and improve for the next time. This process is of a redundant nature, but everyone understands it is part of improving specific skills.

Use the following checklist to verify the audience's point of view:

- Did you tell the audience at an initial phase what you will talk about and how much time you will take (if these two things are not 100% clear)?
- Did you clarify the purpose of the talk (if it is not 100 % clear)?
- The line and blocking of content and timing was expected to be optimal for the view of the listener
- Did you provide a summary at the end of the presentation?
- Did the audience clearly understand the main issues in the presentation?
- And the bottom line: Did the audience find the presentation interesting?

If you answer all these questions with a yes, then you may conclude that the given information was demanded and highly appreciated. The communication was positive, with an interactive information exchange, and a learning process occurred.

7.2 Person-to-Person Communication

Communication between two persons is the most common situation, where each focuses on the other, Fig. 7.3. This is also a

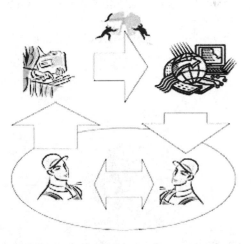

Figure 7.3 Person-to-person communication.

complex situation, where one does not want to persuade the other by pushing arguments in an overconvincing way. If this is done, it will lead to a situation in which the other part becomes defensive and stops providing inputs.

An alternative is to listen to the other person's arguments and opinions and then to use them as a basis for creating your own arguments that are further developed toward your direction of argument. This seems complicated, but the following images will clarify the process of arguing in a constructive way. A real-life conversation is naturally more complex but may include the following moments:

7.2.1 *The Fast Presentation*

A fast presentation is often referred to as an *elevator presentation*, because if you meet someone in the elevator there is time only for a short interaction of one to three minutes, during which you have to provide the other person with enough information about essential matters, as illustrated in Fig. 7.4.

A one-minute presentation can be found on the web pages of fairly big companies. This is a strategy used to provide the reader or listener with essential information. The idea is to create interest in a very short time period, since it is generally known that people do not have time to go through the often too massive information flow available on the Internet.

Five sentences will provide the reader with an easy, understandable introduction to a company in less than a minute. The

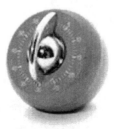

Figure 7.4 A time-dependent presentation requires you to control the time.

core information in those five sentences about the company has to be informative:

- Name and location
- Business
- Products and/or services
- Core function
- Offering to the customer

Here's an example of the structure:

- "Company name" is Eastern Asia's leading player in ...
- The company specializes in managing, developing, and increasing the efficiency of ... in the private/public sector.
- We offer all types of services, from ... to ...
- However, our core strength focuses on ...
- This is we mean by ..., and that is what allows us to ...

Here's an example of a company presentation:

Wide Management is one of the South Asia's leading players in service management. The company specializes in managing, developing, and increasing the efficiency of service functions in offices, properties, production facilities, and the public sector.

We offer all types of services, from running staff canteens and instrument calibration to leasing administration, technical safety solutions, and optimization of premises. However, our core strength lies in developing and managing service functions in new and more efficient ways. This is what we mean by intelligent service, and that is what allows us to guarantee our customers constant improvements in results.

A one-minute presentation can, of course, also be used for personal presentations, such as your home page, social media page, or simply your curriculum vitae (CV). The organization is the same strategic construction of sentences as in the previous example. The structure can be used for organizations as well as interest groups and individuals who want to present short and effective core information.

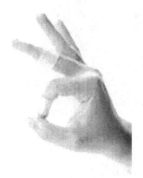

Figure 7.5 A presentation of yourself.

Here is an example of a personal presentation, Fig. 7.5, using the same five-sentence structure:

My name is Ms. Sandra Bullit, a highly skilled competence within service management. I have during the past five years specialized in managing, developing, and increasing the efficiency of service functions in offices, properties, production facilities, and the public sector.

I can offer all types of services, from running staff canteens and instrument calibration to leasing administration, technical safety solutions, and optimization of premises. However, my core strength lies in developing and managing service functions in new and more efficient ways. This is what I mean by intelligent service, and that is what allows me to guarantee my future employer constant improvements in results.

Now, what about designing a one-minute presentation where you present yourself to the managing director of a known and established organization. The presentation should naturally involve your strengths and knowledge. I would not, in this case, recommend that the presentation involve general skills. However, the tradition is often set by the reader and his or her preferences. Therefore, you can present traditional knowledge often obtained from university. This exercise will not cause you any problems, but please note that it is wise to be thoughtful before you make a short, impulsive statement or presentation, whether oral or written.

7.3 Body Language

The science of nonverbal communication, or body language, has attracted remarkable interest during the past decade. Interest has also increased due to academic research considering body language as a multidisciplinary area in order to establish the validity of certain common behaviors.

The science of body language involves the study of a person's:

- facial expressions;
- gestures;
- kinetics (how the body is moved);
- body distance;
- touching and relation to other objects;
- posture; and
- emotions.

Even a person's clothing may be of interest in finding out how:

- the person thinks;
- what his or her intentions are; and
- whether his or her statements are true.

Understanding the behavior of the body is an additional benefit. For a person who wants to really interact with others and learn how to make use of communication abilities, a study of people's nonverbal expressions is required. Whether the aim is to understand friends or classmates or prepare for upcoming job interviews, being able to read a person's intentions can provide a powerful advantage.

Studying your friends' faces when communicating with them is a good opportunity to try to judge their intentions and to follow up your reasoning to determine whether you were right in your assumptions. It may also be of interest to study people talking in front of an audience and learn how they behave when communicating. Are there signs of nervousness or stress? Is the behavior before and after the presentation different? Of course, how a person behaves is most essential. This can be easily detected by asking a friend to focus on your behavior when you talk in front of a group. Or you can videotape yourself and learn about your specific behavior. This will give you an increased understanding about you as an individual and how your behavior changes during stress, etc.

You can learn more about body language by reading scientific articles or popular books available in the library.

7.4 Aim of a Presentation

Why do you put in a lot of time to create a presentation on a subject that you are maybe not comfortable with? In many situations, when someone expects you to make such a presentation, for example, about the company, the quarterly income budget, or simply a course at the university, there is a need to know the expectations with regard to the outcome. Well, the simple reason is that this is part of your expectations or included in your job description. The presentation might also be requested by a person of a higher rank in the organization, for example, your boss.

On the other hand, you may give a presentation about yourself and your prior experience in certain matters during an interview. Your first contact with the human resources (HR) personnel of a company when you are applying for your dream job may start with the following statement by the HR personnel:

> "Welcome to our company. We have now presented our internal organization and the vacancy position that you have applied for. Let us know more about you and why you believe you are the man/woman for this job."

Now your show begins. With delicacy and enthusiasm, and as you have done this presentation hundreds of times, you start to talk about yourself and your university life with authority, followed by your prior work experience, probably at the campus café or even at the reception of a local hotel between semesters.

Always keep in mind that however good or bad you think the presentation is, it is not you who will judge the result. A presentation can be disastrous according to you, but a month later, someone might call you up and ask about the product you presented, leading to an order for the company. Or a presentation can be a success according to you, where the audience applauded and seemed very satisfied, but a week later, nobody might remember the content you worked so hard to communicate.

The aim of a presentation is to communicate with the audience. The communicated message should start an internal process in the listener, for example, "How well can the message in this presentation help me further develop my expectations and solve my problems?"

The way you present information and your ability to communicate it in an engaging form will provide grounds for the listener to receive and further process the information. Of course, the time available for the listener to receive the content is also crucial due to many reasons. If the listener is tired or hungry or there are external disturbances, for example, a noisy industrial environment, perception is not the best.

My best advice to you for such a complex situation where input constraints often are not given is to:

- always be prepared to give a presentation, of yourself, your company, etc.;
- try to adapt the content to the audience's expectations;
- have a reasonable time frame;
- focus on the main message; and
- provide your contact information if someone want to contact you in the future.

The main thing is to learn about the field objectives in the presentation. Use the available technical support that will increase the clarity of the message of the presentation. Include time for some short questions related to your presentation. Also, be dynamic during the presentation and, if necessary, make small adjustments.

Always be prepared to make a presentation but be aware of questions that may arise in related fields.

Chapter 8

Personality: A Student's Best-Acquired Characteristic

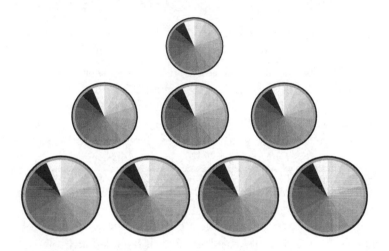

As a student, your own driving force is to be aware of and understand your own behavior. Further, it is also essential for you to estimate how other people will judge your behavior.

8.1 How to Communicate Personality

You have probably read or heard about a person who enters a room and everyone is quiet, eagerly waiting to listen to what he or she

Mastering Technical Communication Skills: A Student's Handbook
Peter Wide
Copyright © 2016 Pan Stanford Publishing Pte. Ltd.
ISBN 978-981-4364-67-6 (Hardcover), 978-981-4364-68-3 (eBook)
www.panstanford.com

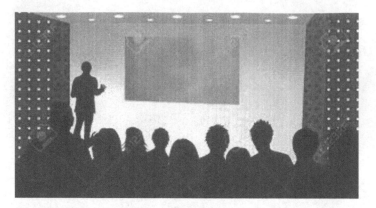

Figure 8.1 Presentation at a meeting with an interested audience.

has to say. You are astonished by the way the person gets all the attention from all "friends" in the room. When the person starts to talk, everyone listens and is engaged in what he or she has to say, as illustrated in Fig. 8.1. There are no questions, objections, or discussions. All listeners just follow the ideas and enthusiastically accept the messages. Everyone in the audience seems to support the persuasive speaker. A student has, of course, something to learn from such "persuasive speakers," whether they are internationally known speakers or just teachers in a school.

There is always time to reflect on your own behavior and how your performance is received. A person's personality, of course, follows him or her, and people can read the conditions (as they are reading an open book) and will continuously judge the person. There are simple dimensions in the human personality, measured by two types of continuum, *extraversion* and *introversion*. These two "opposites" are seen as a branch of psychology that deals with an individual's personality and differences. The field relates to the science of personality psychology.

A person's personality is related to a group of characteristic sets of behaviors that he or she exhibits in different situations:

- When applying for a job
- When working in teams
- When understanding other people's actions

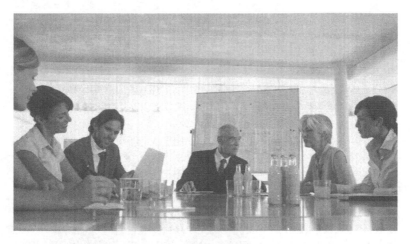

Figure 8.2 An ongoing meeting in a conference room.

For a young individual, it is of great benefit to understand how the personality is used in different situations and to foresee the behavior in a group, when working in a team with a number of different personalities that may cooperate in a certain way. Also it may be of interest to combine different personalities into a working group that has to act as an effective team. Often these challenges are tested when different personalities in a team are going to deliver results within a certain time period, something that frequently happens in business organizations, for example in a meeting as shown in Fig. 8.2.

If you are in a situation in which there is a problem to cooperate with a specific person, for example, in a study group at the university or in high school, there is an important step to identify the properties and learn why this cooperation, sequence, or situation is not working well. Do the personalities differ, for example, is an extrovert person with an assertive manner trying to convince an introvert person by arguing or discussing in the classroom? Or is the problem related to some old diversity of opinion, and what then is the underlying factor? The introvert person may be trying to argue but in a more reserved manner. Since such people may not have the interest or ability to enter a discussion, the situation may be strained. Their personalities may seem to be more reserved and less outgoing, but they still have comments to make.

Both extrovert and introvert personalities are important to make use of the full flavor of competence and cooperative abilities when forming a team, whether in business or in a study task at school. People who do not come into the limelight have to work together with people who love to talk and be the center of attention. All these personalities must be respected in a discussion or a team to achieve the best-possible outcome.

As a useful exercise, it will be of interest to determine your own personal character and reflect over your own behaviors in different situations.

You can ask friends or people who know you about your personality and try to determine the strong and weak parts of your behaviors (as they experience it). This understanding can be of use in situations in which you need to understand how different personalities can strengthen or weaken a discussion, joint working task, or organization.

The following general questions may be of help when estimating your behaviors in conjunction with interactions with other people:

- Do you start a discussion with unknown people (a single person or a group)?
- How do you behave when entering a room where people are standing in many different small groups, each group being involved in an ongoing discussion?
- Do you tremble when facing an audience during a presentation?
- Do you plan a task well in advance, or do you wait for it to resolve as usual in the end at delivery?
- Do you feel stressed about a meeting and worry about the outcome, or do you feel secure and confident?
- Do you like to socialize, or do you prefer fewer social activities?
- Do you have a number of acquaintances or just a few close friends?
- Do you like to talk and be engaged in discussions, or do you just listen and keep your questions and opinions to yourself?
- Do you ask questions after a meeting or lecture, or do you just feel comfortable to listen to an ongoing Q&A discussion?

Try to answer these questions, but also estimate by a simple judgment the results from your friends, and also your foes. You may get some interesting results when comparing yourself with friends and people you do not like.

Remember that all levels between the two extremes of extrovert and introvert personalities are needed in a social activity, and a combination of these personalities in a group, a team, or just a relationship can achieve successful actions and outputs.

As a student learning about behavior, remember one single statement:

You are the person you are!

Probably you are a person with pros and cons but most likely with a preponderance of advantages in individual experience.

There is, however, a tendency to concentrate, during a communication, on the cons, leading to a defensive attitude when entering a discussion. However, everyone, also the presumptive people you have to meet, has a certain amount of uncertainty. Many of the strong and communicative people I have met on different occasions have, at first sight, a negative charisma, probably because their behavior give a charismatic message that they exhibit a secure and convenient feeling of controlling the conversation and mastering the communication. This was, however, completely wrong, since those people have developed a way of thinking and a strategy around such situations. The most impressive meetings are when the person is not even aware of the fact that he or she is controlling the situation. The arguments and facts in the discussion were provided with a sense of humility, but the final result was the opposite—complete success in having all the information and decisions made in controlling the expected direction of the discussion. I asked one of these people, who has the ability to successfully communicate, what the secret solutions are. He just answered that this was achieved by plain, simple training for communicating with people in general. By using this built-up strategy to train to daily communicate and to explore the fine-tuned advantages to achieve, in whatever discussion, provides him with a sincere feeling of satisfaction. This strategy drives him to learn to be more convincing and develop his ability to control the discussion. Developing the ability to successful communicate a message will, at the end, most likely provide the person with an advantage.

However, a general mistake is to underestimate the communicating partner, and this judgment may lead to a negative outcome of a first meeting or discussion. Remember that an interaction with another person also provides him or her with an opinion about you. This opinion once settled is often hard to change or even smoothly redirect.

There seems to be some truth in the following statement:

Every part in an interaction between humans will teach something, whether positive or negative.

8.2 Personal Dynamics

In the old Indian tradition, there has been an understanding of the universe and the humans' place in the world. The traditional teaching by Native American elders was that wherever you are staying in the world, you are in the center of the universe. Even if you have traveled for many days, you will still be in the center of universe. However far you go, you will still be able to observe the earth equidistant around you in all directions as a circle. This observation will, of course, be more effective if you are located in a higher place such as a mountaintop. Then you may notice that wherever you are, the sky stretches over you in all directions.

Native Americans refer to this tradition as the understanding of our place in the universe and the constant presence of the Circle of Life.

This view of Native Americans will also help students find guidance in situations in which they may ask themselves about the meaning of an interview or why they have to go through a boring course at the university. If everyone is the in center of the universe, why do many of us undergo hours as passive participants and only notice events that happen around us day after day?

Instead, we should have the ability to act as if we were in the center of this interview or that course at the university and that these events are especially created for us and our intention to be the center.

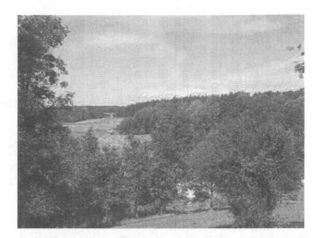

Figure 8.3 A feeling of taking care of the moment – CARPE DIEM.

We could then literally be in the center of the universe and become an active part in the events. This attitude will then be reflected in our facial expressions and body language, definitively declaring that we have an aura. The attitude will clearly show that we can actively take part in the events, discussions, and communication and provide arguments with self-confidence and self-esteem.

As an outcome of this exercise, my sincere intention is, of course, to make students more independent and active and including them as human beings in order to take part in the dynamic activities that always will occur, as described in Fig. 8.3. I would like to highlight that students are not only learning and arguing but also continuously interacting constructively in learning situations. Positive communication should occur, where young people do not leave a lecture at the university without asking needed questions that probably would clarify the whole situation. I would like to see young people going to their first interview with a smile on their face and confident about the meeting. Because they are, each and every one of them, at that moment, in their individual mind, in the center of the universe. This is their belief and a thought in their brain. That is why it is worth keeping this feeling and making a positive impression from it. *Carpe diem*!

8.3 Social Behavior

According to *The Oxford Dictionary of English*, the phrase "social behavior" means "the way in which one acts or conducts oneself, especially towards others."

The ability to attract and fascinate listeners in a meeting or a big audience is, of course, related to how a person is able to compel his or her attractiveness or charm in order to inspire devotion in others.

We have probably all met people who are engaging, enthusiastic, and convincing when talking, for example, a teacher or a politician who really fascinates listeners.

These people have a natural talent for communicating with others. They have a social charisma that attracts other people with their social behavior.

Whether it is a natural gift or a talent to learn the rules of social behavior, it is, for sure, an argument in favor of learning how to communicate with people and be aware of one's own social behavior. The main question is, then, how is my behavior perceived by others?

Training to communicate socially involves understanding your own behavior and what signals you send out to other people. A person's social behavior is of great importance to understand and determine your own and the person's social charisma. Find your own strengths and limitations.

There are a number of actions that strengthen social behavior. These actions can, of course, be learned and implemented as natural behavior:

- Be a good listener when people talk.
- Provide constructive comments in a discussion.
- Provide informative and relevant information.
- Have also a sense of humor in discussions.
- Show empathy, when needed.
- Be determined in communicating a specific issue.
- Be strong-minded but also listening when you are arguing for an opinion.
- Be reasonable when judging people.
- Be humble in interacting with other people.
- Evaluate other people's arguments.

The main and final outcome of this section is that whatever type of personality you meet in your social network, there is a need to *always take care of your social contacts, get rid of negative people and strengthen the ones who give you positive feedback. Be an active but responsible part of social media, like LinkedIn and Facebook.*

Social behavior in a group or team is an important aspect. To build up a team that will create a joint competence base and each member's skills, experience, and personality will complement those of the other members is a delicate job. Normally, there are not a lot of choices to be made, but usually there are a number of people available to join a team. The aim is to get a group of competencies that complement each other in knowledge and are fitting in the group atmosphere, goals, and social engagement. In a small group everyone is expected to contribute with his or her skills and interact with coworkers in a manner that fosters creativity and innovative thinking and focuses on results to achieve the expected goals.

Many complex organizations are structured with an advanced connection of people of different ages, cultural and ethnical backgrounds, and knowledge. A knowledge-based organization if managed right, is the ultimate working place, where outcomes and deliverables are created through a genuine working collaboration.

On the other hand, if not managed right and with unclear directives and working frames, things may also go wrong, with disputes and other personal problems in the group.

8.4 The Personal Brand

To feel your personal brand is to know yourself, how others see you, and the realization that you can control this. This is a critical factor for a successful career. It is just a matter of understanding your personality and to communicate it to relevant people.

How do you want to be perceived?

Think about how you want to be perceived by others. Get an insight into what factors determine what other people will experience when meeting you in different situations, for example, in a meeting, a class, or a job interview.

This concept can be seen as a preventive action to get yourself an insight into how you are expected to be perceived by others, and

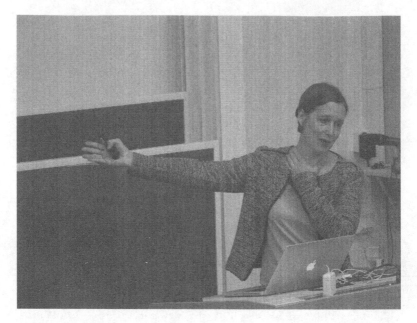

Figure 8.4 A person's personality brand is a valuable asset.

you can train yourself and also experience it. This way, it will not be too much of a surprise when you enter a meeting and interact with other people.

It may also be of interest to learn by observing other people and studying their behaviors during meetings or even on television. Think about what makes these people successful and why you admire their personalities.

To build up an individual personality character that can be used as a personal brand is of importance, but it is really just a matter of self-awareness. A personal brand is to learn to know yourself and your strengths and weaknesses and to communicate these properties to other people.

A personal brand is not just a buzzword for bloggers, entrepreneurs, or celebrities, Fig. 8.4. Actually, it involves a number of abilities:

First, and most important, is how you look at yourself. Your personal brand is also about your profile of competence, experience, and personality. One could say that it is about putting into words personal qualities that are difficult to put into a curriculum vitae (CV). Often qualities like personal strength, commitment, courage, and curiosity are key factors as determinants of success.

A personal brand is relevant for everyone, especially for a student who is aiming to enter a career after education. The key issue is to explain and communicate the personal brand and how it is perceived by others.

Next is to take control over your personal brand and to modify how you are perceived by other people. An illustrative example is to modify the properties by which young students are perceived when a certain style is convenient in school. Students may be casually dressed, with a specific appearance in class, reticent in discussions, and not active in social events. When finishing school, a thoughtful approach is required to deal with the preferences that exist outside school. It is important that the former student be able to highlight those qualities in him or her that would make him or her a good employee in a specific company in a specific position. Maybe some added features are needed when changing from student life to work life, such as creativity, ambition, and teamwork ability, which are qualities that maybe are not too required in the educational phase.

No matter which direction you intend to choose in a career, it is important to reflect on qualities that other people notice as strengths and to ensure that these are communicated to people who are going to assess your personality. Students have, in general, good self-awareness, but they have to adapt it to different arenas, like academia or business. Some students may be too shy in using their strengths and need to dare to communicate their personal brands.

Here is a structured path to establish your personal brand:

- **Find out how other people perceive you.** Have the courage to ask others how they perceive you as a person.
- **Compile your brand.** Get an insight into how those around you perceive you.

- **Remember that your personal brand is fresh information.** Update the content frequently.
- **Direct your personal brand to your aims.** Remember, this may vary during your change of direction in career development.

Chapter 9

Future Aspects: The Time a Student Is Active

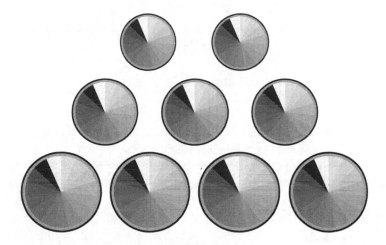

Predicting the future world situation in the coming 30 to 40 years is always hazardous. The development of society from now to 2050 will, for sure, be as revolutionary as we can expect it to be. However, we can get an idea of the development in 2050 if we look at history 30 or 40 years back in time. The change in society and how technological improvements will affect us highlight a key problem: *It is difficult to*

Mastering Technical Communication Skills: A Student's Handbook
Peter Wide
Copyright © 2016 Pan Stanford Publishing Pte. Ltd.
ISBN 978-981-4364-67-6 (Hardcover), 978-981-4364-68-3 (eBook)
www.panstanford.com

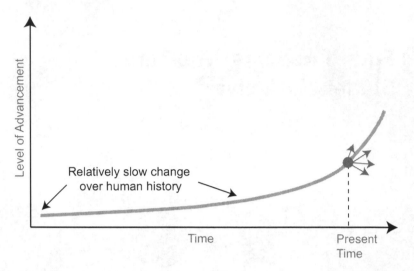

Figure 9.1 Predicting the future is difficult.

imagine the future. What we can do, however, is make the best of it and try to adapt to future developments (Fig. 9.1).

Science fiction literature of the previous two centuries predicted amazing things, for example, going to the moon, exploring the subsea, using fast transportation, and talking to each other over long distances. These activities became a common part of our lives. However, these worked well when the pace of change was slow. But over the past few decades, the rate of social and technological change has increased, and evolution is grinding to a halt as people are hitting the limits of their imagination and foresight. The moment where change occurs so rapidly that we cannot imagine what will happen is amazing. The question is whether humans, with all their limitations, will be able to fully join the fast evolution.

9.1 The World When You Will Retire

The world in the future will, for sure, be something else compared to what we experience today. No one can imagine how we will fit into that future society, and it is meaningless to guess, at least if we are not sure of the progress shown in Fig. 9.1.

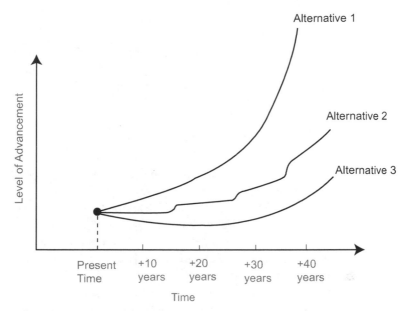

Figure 9.2 One trend indicating development in the next 30–40 years.

But if we expect that development will continue like today, the trend can be as shown in Fig. 9.2.

Further, if we estimate the positive development trend to be like it was in the last 30–40 years, we may interpolate the curve, e.g. alternative 1, in the future, as shown in Fig. 9.2.

However, if the future trend will be as illustrated in alternative 2, then we will experience different paradigm shifts in the society, that will mainly cause an increasing step wise result. Step wise advancements may for example be improvements in climate change, environment and cure of diseases, and also new solutions in energy sector, effective medical treatments, drugs or an improved social interaction by the use of internet.

There may also be a negative or small social and technology developments in the advancement, e.g. alternative 3, with no or maybe a small advancement in the coming 30-40 years, e.g. due to economic or conflict reasons.

What will the trend be then in the coming years that will have a major effect on a student of today?

Will the development change our personalities? Probably, because the way we act, behave, and interact will change over time. When looking in the mirror, we may just accept the fact that the best personal requirements when our grandparents were applying for jobs are not the same as today's.

Some trends are more highlighted than others:

- Information flow will need to be handled in more optimally than it is today. This means that the more intelligent and powerful the computers that are developed, the more the information handling that we can manage.
- Information search, collection, analysis, and presentation will probably be some of the most important factors that will help us manage jobs of the future.
- We also have to learn these advanced skills when making a career, in the same manner as our grandparents learned how to manage the first computers.

This evolution is considered transformative when a myriad of data streams, impulses, desires, and even consciousnesses will interact with us as we navigate multiple worlds. The virtual societies are places where we enter social transformations and live in besides our real world. As avatars in, for example, a "second life," we can live an active life as virtual entrepreneurs.

9.2 Your Place in the Development Phase

The place for a student who will earn a university degree within a year may look frightening but also challenging. Is it possible to join activities in society and also learn about all the new technology that continuously will pop up in life and benefit your career?

Future jobs will probably be less connected to a place or location. Work can partly be performed from a home office. There will be new possibilities of innovation and product design using the Internet. New economies will grow that are not attached to specific countries. The focus on increasing human performance and making the elderly enjoy life by increasing their perception will create jobs. The fact that people will get healthier and older and a generation of retired people will look for new ways of entertaining, traveling, and enjoyable experiences will create a global market.

The new era of individual requirements is not fully considered by the market today, but the expectation of a growing global industry era has just begun.

9.3 Taking Care of Yourself

What is the expectation from a student of today in these coming decades?

Well, there is no expectation, at least not from society.

However, the message in this book is to plan for tomorrow and be aware of all the challenges that will be present.

Every student's has his or her own path of planning a career and getting a nice, enjoyable, but also achievable and expected life. A student's language skills and choices of courses and degrees by themselves will not make the student happy. But if these can help provide the student with a career that will increase his or her satisfaction and make him or her enjoy life, it may be worth it.

The final message of this book is just a simple recommendation to go out into the world with a spirit of joy, knowing that you have the basic knowledge to progress and take part in the development.

It does not matter where you come from; the only thing that matters is where you are going.

Index